Freedom and Independence

RETAINING THE MIND SERIES: BOOK TWO

WILLIAM EMMETT WALSH, MD

ISBN: 978-1-7346396-2-9 (paperback)

LCCN:
Edited by Peter Bergh
Typeset and Cover Design by www.ebookbook.com

Printed in the United States of America

Other books by Dr. Walsh

Escape From Dementia, Retaining the Mind Series, Book 1, Revision 2

How I Recovered From Dementia: Retaining the Mind Series: Book 1, Revised

Retaining the Mind: How the Foods We Eat Affect Our Brain

Home Allergies: Don't Let Your Home Make You Sick

Food Allergies: The Complete Guide to Understanding and Relieving Your Food Allergies

The Food Allergy Book: The Foods That Cause You Pain and Discomfort and How to Take Them out of Your Diet

Treating Food Allergy, My Way: Exploring the Most Important Food Allergies, Second Edition

Treating Sinus, Migraine, and Cluster Headaches, My Way: An Allergist's Approach to Headache Treatment

Treating Food Allergy, My Way: Exploring the Most Important Food Allergies

Acknowledgments

I thank my patients who so kindly and graciously showed me that our modern diet is poisonous. I thank Meredithe and my son, Bill, for eating the foods I prepared while I learned how to prepare a diet that reverses dementia. I especially thank those who hear me and read my books because I write for you.

Contents

Foreword

Freedom and Independence is the second book of my *Retaining the Mind* series. I titled it *Freedom and Independence* because I love to be free and I love to be independent. Free to go to church or the movies, to drive three hundred miles to see a friend, or to write a book that helps others.

Our modern diet tries to take away our freedom and independence by making us sick, including diseases of the heart, lung, and intestine as well as infectious diseases. It assists the growth of our cancers and encourages autoimmune diseases like multiple sclerosis, lupus, and rheumatoid arthritis. It handicaps our thinking and increases our depressions and anxieties.

I suffer from Alzheimer's and Parkinson's dementias, a not uncommon combination. I know that these dementias arise from what we eat and drink because our modern diet is poisonous. Resisting this poisoning helps preserve our freedom and independence.

After having diagnosed and treated diet-caused diseases for years, I know that dementias are simple diseases, and I want you to understand this simplicity. If I teach you about them, you will relieve some of the burdens a poor diet exerts on our bodies and minds.

This year, I revised and published the first book in my *Retaining the Mind* series: *Escape From Dementia.* With *Freedom* and *Independence,* I am publishing again. *Escape From Dementia* concentrates on treating mild forms of dementia; *Freedom and Independence* focuses on controlling dementia as it becomes more severe. If dementia threatens you or a loved one, these books will show you how to reverse this brain-destroying disease.

I want you to know that our foods and beverages are dangerous. Knowing this danger and counteracting it prevented my falling into mental deterioration and death. May my words do the same for you.

Treating illness by improving diet fascinates me, and I can teach you how to do the same. A better understanding of our foods and beverages will help you subdue dementia that otherwise would be pitiless.

Before following my diet, please have your medical caregivers evaluate your condition. Other illnesses can behave like diet-caused diseases but need different treatment, so be sure you do not suffer from one of them before following my suggestions.

1

Simplifying Dementia

The Dementias Are Simple Diet-Caused Diseases

Once you understand the dementias, you will realize that they are simple diseases. Unfortunately, many people do not know that dementia is a simple disease; instead, they believe that dementia is too complicated to understand or reverse, so they do not know how to defeat it. I will try to show you how to both understand and reverse dementia.

Many treatment suggestions promoted by skilled and knowledgeable teachers—such as mind and body exercise—help treat the dementias; please do not ignore their advice. My focus is on careful food and beverage selection and preparation to reverse dementia. This diet selection is at least as crucial as mind and body exercise in treating dementia and maybe more critical because dementia reversal occurs only with this diet change.

Dementia From Excess Aging Chemicals

Dementias arise from two sources in the foods that we eat and the beverages we drink. Our overuse of specific flavorful food chemicals is one source. As I have already discussed, these chemicals are harmless if we take them in the amount we tolerate. These chemicals are the simple sugars fructose and galactose, the amino acid MSG, and the food acids associated with citrus. We already covered these food chemicals in *Escape From Dementia*, and I will review them again and add to your knowledge of them in this book.

I will try to show you how to understand dementia and the food chemicals that cause it. Then you can decide if you want to exercise careful diet selection and preparation so you can continue to enjoy an alert mind.

Dementia From Vegetables and Fruits

Because of their chemical defenses, our vegetables and fruits participate in causing sickness, including dementia. They use toxins (poisons) that they produce to repel the predators that would destroy them. Unfortunately, when we eat plant-derived foods, we eat these same poisons. To avoid the poisonous effects of these toxins, organisms as primitive as jellyfish and as complicated as humans have a barrier protecting the brain from them—the blood–brain barrier. Unfortunately, as we age, this barrier in many of us becomes far less effective, allowing food poisons to slip through and attack and damage the brain, the damage eventually destroying the brain.

Repairing the barrier and eating foods without toxins would cure dementia. However, we do not know how to fix the barrier, and we cannot take away from plants their toxins; they must have toxins for self-defense. Mold, insects, or animals would destroy any food plants that did not have toxins before we had the chance to eat them or drink their juices. We can still eat these vegetables and fruits and resist these diseases by choosing our diet carefully and preparing food in methods that reduce the toxins we would otherwise consume.

From the information I have discussed, we now have a simple explanation of this brain-destroying disease. Toxins cause dementia by damaging the brain after penetrating through the damaged blood–brain barrier.

Different Dementias Have Common Causes

The various dementias like Alzheimer's, Parkinson's, and Lewy body dementias are all diet-caused diseases, with the difference between dementias arising because each attacks a different area in the brain. This similar cause simplifies dementia because we do not need to learn various reasons for each dementia. The area of the brain damaged by dementia is probably the area that malfunctioning genes control. We will probe deeper into this gene control in future chapters.

I use the terms "dementia," "dementias," or "the dementias" to discuss the group of diseases that include dementias like Alzheimer's or Parkinson's diseases. As I discuss each dementia, I will call it by its name, as in "Alzheimer's dementia" or "Alzheimer's disease."

You may want to explore further many of the statements I will make in this book. To guide you in your research, as these articles guided me, I am providing links to articles with this information. By including these references I am not indicating that they are the best articles to use in understanding what I am discussing, only that most of them are relatively recent and their content attracted me.

https://tinyurl.com/y32xlxov

https://www.verywellhealth.com/what-is-the-blood-brain-barrier-3980707

2

I Want to Help

S ome of my friends suffer from failing eyesight that prevents them from watching TV or reading a book. Other friends suffer from impaired hearing. Their impaired sight and hearing may arise from damage to the nerves of sight and hearing from the toxins in our diet. When I suggest changing their diets to determine if their sight and hearing will stop deteriorating and hopefully even recover, they brush off the suggestion. I must sound nutty; how could their favorite foods and beverages hurt their eyes and ears?

One of these friends with hearing difficulty sat beside me at a church service. His right ear, the ear closest to me, was completely deaf, and the hearing in his left ear was so weak that he could hardly hear me, even when he turned his whole body to bring his left ear close to me so I could talk directly into that ear. His inability to hear the ceremony saddened him so much that he left the service early before I could suggest a diet change that might save and—at least partially—restore his hearing.

Was I right in suspecting his foods and beverages cause his deafness? It is more than a faint possibility. If I start losing my sight or hearing, I will become even more compulsive in reducing the toxins in my diet.

Other friends have lost so much memory that they cannot remember recent events. I doubt they are aware that their diet may be at fault: The afflicted are the last to realize that they have dementia. Whether or not they suspect it, dementia could be degrading their memories, sight, and hearing.

Can I force them to listen to me? Of course not. I can only help those who will listen.

I Want to Help

Experts call many modern diets healthy, but my diet goes beyond these other diets. My diet attacks and reverses dementia. It contradicts some present-day advice on treating this condition, which leads astray those who could benefit from a low-toxin diet—my diet controls and reverses dementia. If people with dementia try my diet, they will find that it brings them enormous rewards. Perhaps it improves sight or hearing for those suffering from damaged nerves of sight and hearing. Or it may return balance when standing or walking to those whose illness brings poor balance, even freeing them from canes or wheelchairs.

Or the reward could be feeling much more alive as they lose the excess weight that threatens them with diabetes, strokes, or heart attacks. Or perhaps the gift is seeing the return of alertness to the face of a loved one.

I am an ordinary man; the illnesses that affect me are diseases that affect many people. My experience tells me that this is true; many people suffer from the same diseases trying to destroy me. If Alzheimer's, Lewy body, or Parkinson's diseases slow their thinking; if their sight, hearing, or balance deteriorate; if they suffer strokes or heart attacks; if depression or anxiety haunts them, my diet resists these maladies. There is a possibility that what they eat and drink shares much of the blame for their misfortune, and diet change may help heal their bodies and minds.

Let Them Try My Diet

If the diet change works, the people following my suggestions will know how to recover from dementia. If it does not work for them, at least they had a chance to try for recovery. It worked in my patients and me; I diagnosed and treated hundreds of food-sensitive patients referred to me by their doctors in my medical practice. Many found great relief from distressing debilities by careful diet choice. Now I suffer from Alzheimer's and Parkinson's dementia, and these diet changes help me.

Knowing that you and others can enjoy the return of sight, hearing, balance, and thinking rewards my writing. Those suffering from damaged nerves should not feel alone. I also suffered this damage. I followed dementia's downward path until I developed severe dementia. My deterioration frightened me into changing my diet; that change returned my ability to think, talk, and write. You or a loved one may find these same rewards by following my diet, and I will be so pleased.

Our Diet's Financial Burden

I often think of how much money society spends diagnosing and treating diet-caused diseases. Judy George in

MedPage Today shares my concerns. She noted that 5.8 million Americans have Alzheimer's disease, and certificates recorded 122,019 deaths from Alzheimer's disease in 2018. Horrible numbers! And these expenses and fatalities will increase as many disease-stricken sufferers become older, a group too numerous for any society to treat.

https://www.medpagetoday.com/neurology/alzheimers disease/85374

But many people can treat themselves—with less expense—at home, at their dining table. Cautious dieting can reverse dementia and restore the good health of the mind and body. My books contain the information they need to reverse this disease.

Although I point out the many women and men harmed by our modern American diet, I do not think of them as a crowd. I think of each individually. My good wishes go to each of them. My concern for them keeps me determined to help them. I want to bring the same improvement I gained—the blessings I received—to those who read my books and hear me speak. I pray that my information helps them leave our diet's destructive path and find the road to health.

These thoughts guide me as I write.

3

A Healthy Diet

The *U.S. News & World Report* (2020) lists the healthiest American diets. They list the Mediterranean Diet number one, the DASH, and the Mayo Clinic (my alma mater) diets in the top five. The *Mediterranean Diet* emphasizes eating fruits, vegetables, whole grains, beans, nuts, legumes, olive oil, and flavorful herbs and spices. It encourages eating fish and seafood several times weekly, and poultry, eggs, cheese, and yogurt in moderation while reserving sweets and red meat for special occasions.

The *DASH Diet* (Dietary Approaches to Stop Hypertension) emphasizes fruits, vegetables, whole grains, lean protein, and low-fat dairy. This diet discourages foods high in saturated fat, such as fatty meats, full-fat dairy foods, tropical oils, and sugar-sweetened beverages and treats.

The Mayo Clinic Diet emphasizes fruit, legumes, vegetables, whole-wheat flour, and wheat bran. It encourages fiber-rich foods such as nuts and beans and heart-healthy fish like salmon, mackerel, and tuna. It also promotes "good" fats, which include avocados, almonds, olives, and walnuts. It avoids saturated fats, trans fats, cholesterol, refined sugar, and excess sodium.

https://health.usnews.com/best-diet/best-diets-overall

Good Diets Fail

These diets are undoubtedly healthy. Those who follow them maintain their health much longer than those who eat our modern unrestricted diet. Many authorities believe that these diets improve health by promoting certain "healthy" foods and beverages and discouraging "unhealthy" foods. I think these authorities are both right and wrong.

The value of these diets lies not in the foods they *promote* but instead in the foods they *discourage*. They avoid consuming certain foods and beverages that contain increased refined sugar and, to some degree, more excess amounts of MSG. In other words, the diets are not healthy because they advocate avoiding certain *foods* but because they advocate avoiding certain food *chemicals*, refined sugar, and MSG. Avoiding these two chemicals slows the onset of dementia and improves the health of the diner. However, as we grow older and more susceptible to diseases like strokes, heart disease, and the mental fog of dementia, these diets fail us. They fail us because they overlook other harmful food chemicals that are as damaging as sugar and MSG.

Looking for Causes of Diseases

When I evaluate ill patients, I look for the cause of their illnesses. I look for the virus causing abdominal discomfort, the germs causing pneumonia, the pollen causing sneezing, and the dust that causes wheezing. I do the same in food-sensitive patients, but I do not look for viruses, bacteria, dust, or mold; I look through the patient's diet for troubling food chemicals. I do not concentrate on the supposedly unhealthy foods and beverages, as I believe they are necessary parts of the diet when the afflicted must avoid excess toxic chemicals. If the diets do not avoid excess food toxins, eating "healthy" foods will not prevent dementia. Instead, the afflicted should reduce the harmful chemicals in foods and drinks instead of worrying about healthy and unhealthy foods.

The Mediterranean, DASH, and Mayo Clinic diets allow their followers to consume excess amounts of galactose, MSG, and citrus acids. These diet chemicals make people sick and ultimately kill them. The experts who developed the diets would limit these destructive food chemicals if they knew their harm. I do not want you to make this error: I want you to know about these dangerous diet chemicals.

Once you learn about them, you can join me in searching for other harmful chemicals. And when you find them, you may be improving the diet I advocate! That's what I did. I found that avoiding refined sugar helped me, but this avoidance did not release me from dementia. I was older, and my dementia was so severe that I needed to find additional causes of my mental deterioration; I needed to limit the other health-stomping, youth-killing chemicals. I found them in foods and beverages that the Mediterranean, DASH, and Mayo Clinic diets do not discourage.

I cannot remain healthy and clear thinking while eating and drinking more of these chemicals than I can metabolize. This excess threatens me with dementia and other common diseases I have mentioned, including strokes, heart attacks, and obesity—and the Alzheimer's and Parkinson's diseases that want to control me.

I have devoted my previous books to this task; I also dedicate this book to this task.

My Diet Is Better

Am I saying that the Mediterranean, Mind, and Mayo Clinic diets are not the best diets, that mine is better? Yes, I am, especially for someone plunging deeply into the dementia swamp. Because these other diets do not limit the intake of many problem food chemicals; they restrict the diet follower's improvement. This defect is significant and leads to false conclusions. The "healthy" diet they study may be destroying the brain, while the subject of the diet experiments continues his diet. A proper diet study would limit or avoid the excessive fructose, MSG, citrus acids, and galactose that I already pointed out in previous books.

Contradicting Diet Experts

I find one question fascinating. How can experts be unaware of the damages caused by these other aging chemicals? They could discover them as I did by asking thousands of food-sensitive patients which foods trouble them. Some of their patients would point out these foods and beverages that cause their distress, and the experts could build more healthful diets.

The experts who developed the Mediterranean, DASH, and Mayo Clinic diets are not the only experts I contradict. I'm afraid I also must disagree with many other knowledgeable and respected experts. They include experts in aging at the National Institute on Aging of the National Institutes of Health. These experts deserve respect for the good they do, but they are wrong in one teaching. Recall their definition of Alzheimer's dementia: They term it "an irreversible, progressive brain disorder that slowly destroys memory and thinking skills, and, eventually, the ability to carry out the simplest tasks." They call it a lethal disease that kills the sufferer.

That is true if sufferers do not know the causes of dementia; this lack of knowledge makes dementia lethal. However, if those with dementia understand their disease, they know it arises from the diet. The right diet changes give them a significant chance to recover from dementia, including Alzheimer's, Parkinson's, and Lewy body diseases. I am recovering from Alzheimer's and Parkinson's diseases and will continue to recover if I choose and prepare my foods carefully.

My Patients Contributed to My Diet

I admit I have two advantages that many of the laboratory scientists involved in diet experiments lack. One advantage occurred in the past, and one appears in the present. The past advantage: As I mentioned, I evaluated and treated hundreds of patients referred to me for suspected food allergies each year for forty years. In most of these cases, my patients suffered not from a food *allergy* but food *sensitivity*. I asked them which foods made them suffer, and they told me. Migraine patients were a good source of this information as many already knew and avoided the foods and beverages causing their painful headaches. I put their knowledge into a diet that avoided the troubling foods and drinks, and the diet helped hundreds of patients.

I eventually figured out that these chemicals also age us. They cause or worsen many diseases. The improved health of my food-sensitive patients attracted many other food-sensitive patients to my medical practice, seeking the same relief. These additional patients gave me even more experience in food chemical-induced food sensitivity. Now I find this diet essential in my recovery from dementia.

My Second Advantage: I Have Alzheimer's Dementia

The second advantage I have over the diet experts is my Alzheimer's dementia. My Alzheimer's disease sometimes transitions to Parkinson's dementia. It gives me a unique insight into these diseases and how to recover from them. When you suffer from an illness, you get to know it intimately. I know dementia intimately.

My Contribution to the Diet

As I mentioned, my diet contribution lies not in identifying the chemicals that age us and cause dementia but in gathering my patients' wisdom and stitching it together into a story that explains how and why the diet works. I spent much time understanding why the diet worked—much time reading hundreds of diet studies. In some reports, the authors point out that excessive amounts of troubling chemicals damage nerves. They also mention that these chemicals age us, prompting me to call them the aging chemicals.

Damage to nerves by these chemicals explains the cause of migraine headaches that I mentioned above. Under the scalp, arteries and nerves travel together in a sheath called the neurovascular bundle. With each heartbeat, arteries continually thump on the nerve that travels next to it as the arteries pulsate (expand and contract with the heartbeat). The pulsation does not trouble the nerves if they are undamaged. However, when the nerves are damaged, the arteries beating on them cause throbbing head pain, the migraine headache.

My diet decreases the amount of nerve-damaging chemicals in our food, allowing the migraine-affected nerves to recover and preventing the throbbing pain of migraine headaches. People suffering from diseases caused by these chemicals owe thanks to my migraine patients' who identified these troubling food chemicals.

Summary

My readers can use my diet to fight many diseases, including strokes, diabetes, heart disease, and mental distress that includes depression. My diet helps me control my dementia, and I want my readers to know how to do the same. With this knowledge, and by following my diet, they can gain the chance to recover their ability to think, plan, and act. I have devoted much effort to spread this information to whoever will hear and read the information I provide. Their recovery is my reward for my work.

4

Food Chemicals Cause Disease

The food chemicals that cause many diseases impact all ages, with the elderly suffering the most as they transition into their fifties and beyond. In my Young Brain / Old Brain chapter of this book, I will further discuss this targeting of seniors and how these chemicals age us. In the following few chapters, I will return to the aging chemicals that turn toxic when we consume more of them than our body's digestive system can handle. Then, I will discuss the toxins in fruits and vegetables.

To remain healthy, we should be cautious about consuming the troubling food chemicals at any stage in life, increasing this caution as we grow older. In my previous books, I discussed many of these food chemicals; this chapter presents a refresher course for those who read the earlier books and a chance to learn more about the troubling chemicals. To those new to this knowledge, I am providing a first-time look at these chemicals. The following are the foods and beverages normal to our body and toxic in excess.

- Refined sugars (fructose)
- Monosodium glutamate (MSG), including
  - o low-calorie sweeteners (LCS)
  - o gluten
- Milk sugar (galactose)
- Citrus acids (including citric, malic, fumaric, succinic, and tartaric acids)

5

Refined Sugar

The information about refined sugar in *Escape From Dementia*, my first book of the *Retaining the Mind series,* is as pertinent today as it was when I published this information in 2016. I will review the information about refined sugar and discuss my experience with it. Following this, I will show you how our knowledge of refined sugar guides us in understanding the dementias. This understanding, and the actions this knowledge suggests, identifies steps to help us preserve our minds and our lives as we recover from many diseases, including dementia.

What Is Refined Sugar?

Refined sugar is the sugar in your sugar bowl or your sweet treats. Called sucrose, it consists of two simple sugars bound together, glucose and fructose. Both are tiny chemicals, each with a skeleton of six carbon atoms. They cannot be absorbed from the intestinal tract and into your body until they separate from each other in the intestines. Once separated, our bodies find glucose useful because every cell absorbs it and with it generates energy. We store the excess glucose as glycogen. Although our bodies find that glucose is no problem, fructose is a problem. Like glucose, our bodies naturally contain fructose and use it to create the energy necessary for life. However, the body can use only limited fructose. When our foods and beverages contain more fructose than we can handle, it troubles us.

Dementia and Refined Sugar

Studies show that consuming excess fructose encourages dementia like Alzheimer's Disease; avoiding this extra fructose delays the onset of dementia. This delay is impressive: A diet change that slows dementia? Many drugs intended to control dementia have failed this task. As I mentioned, the Mediterranean, MIND, and Mayo Clinic diets discourage consuming excess sugar, explaining why experts regard them as healthy. Even though they prolong the life of the afflicted, which is a remarkable accomplishment, these diets fail in another task. They do not reverse dementia, and this failure forces the afflicted to continue to suffer dementia until it kills them. A healthy diet should limit all the destructive chemicals in our diet; this limitation will stop dementia's progression, permit recovery from this horror, and save the diet follower's life.

The Fructose–Glucose Ratio

I do not believe anyone knows why the body tolerates so little fructose, but these are my thoughts. Nature is conservative; it does not prepare us to handle large amounts of food chemicals if we do not need this ability. As our foods and beverages naturally contain only a limited amount of fructose, nature gave us only one organ to metabolize fructose—the liver. Stated in another way: the genes that determine our health can handle only small amounts of fructose.

We still cannot handle large amounts of fructose in modern life as our livers are still the only organ to clean up the massive doses we consume in sweet treats. These treats flood the body with fructose, and this sugar in excess causes obesity and other health problems.

To understand how this obesity occurs, assume that our bodies maintain a ratio of fructose to glucose. I will arbitrarily pick one fructose molecule in our bodies for every five molecules of glucose. The plants and animals we eat have this same fructose–glucose ratio. During winter's cold winds or summer's dry spells, the times of starvation, our glucose level falls because we are starving. But, even in famine, the body tries to maintain the same fructose level because this level of fructose is necessary for life. If the fructose level decreases, our metabolism makes more fructose from glucose, attempting to maintain the usual 1:5 ratio of fructose–glucose, but the ratio is no longer 1:5.

The body recognizes this increased fructose ratio, understands that it signals starvation, and tells the body to conserve energy. The body lowers its use of glucose for energy and uses the excess fructose from the diet to convert food calories to fat. We store the fat in the abdomen and the arteries, including those of the brain and heart. The obesity resulting from eating and drinking excess fructose (which affects a high percentage of our population) promotes strokes, heart attacks, diabetes, dementia, and many other diseases that fill our hospital beds and empty our wallets.

Our Modern Diet and the Ratio

Farmers have learned to grow plants with high fructose contents because plants with more fructose taste sweeter and sell better. It is the sweetness of cookies, pies, donuts, and ice cream and we drink it in fructose-sweetened beverages.

The fructose–glucose ratio is my invention. I use it to explain why the body goes into starvation mode when there is no starvation—when there is plenty of high-fructose sugar in our food. This starvation-among-plenty causes the 3Ds: Disease, Dementia, and Death.

The Fat Control System

I continue to avoid the sweet treats that contain excess fructose, following the diet I started following years ago when I weighed 248 pounds. My weight at first decreased to 145 pounds, and I mean 145 pounds. Not 143 to 150 pounds. Not even 142 to 152 pounds. Every morning and many evenings, I weighed myself, and the pointer on the scale always rested on the slash marking 145 pounds. Consistently, day after day, month after month. It might move from the left side of the slash pointing to 145 or the right side or stay right in the middle, but it always stayed at 145 pounds. Amazing! I had lost more than 100 pounds, and my weight was being maintained, not by me, but by my body's fat control system. I stayed at that weight, no matter how much I ate.

I named this system the "fat regulatory system," but I am renaming it since I do not know if anybody else has noticed this system. I decided to retire the term "regulatory" and replace it with "control," a more comfortable word to say and remember.

As you can suspect, this strict weight control exerted by my body, with no dieting by me except avoidance of the troubling chemicals, astounded me. No matter how much or how little I ate, I weighed 145 pounds. Except—you knew there would be an except—if I strayed from my diet. Then the pointer moved to 148 or 149 pounds, alerting me to the need to hurry back to my diet. I did, and I returned to 145 pounds. With further slow weight loss, I now weigh 135 pounds.

I like this system: It protects me from obesity. I do not want to suffer from dementia's dulled intellect, be blocked from driving a car, or be locked in some memory unit. With someone cleaning my bed and me after a poor night of sleep. Ugh!

Olive Oil and the Fat Control System

Then came a drop in my weight, from 145 pounds to 140 pounds. Like my 100-pound loss, this decreased weight happened suddenly, from 145 pounds to 140 pounds. And the pointer points to 140 pounds now, morning and evening. Not 137 to 143 pounds. One hundred forty pounds right on the slash mark pointing to the number "140." My total weight loss is now more than one hundred pounds.

I know the reason for the five-pound weight loss. In reading about diets, I noticed some diets did not use olive oil, and I decided to avoid this oil. Four days after I stopped using olive oil, five pounds dropped off the scale. I had been carrying five pounds of the bloat because of the olive oil. I had used it liberally because the "best" diets regard it as healthy. I am sure it is a healthy oil but perhaps not for those who, like me, have a severe degree of dementia.

So, the fat control system may hold your weight at a healthy level if you avoid fructose sweets, but you can still bloat because of the other food chemicals. Imagine, I was unknowingly carrying around five extra pounds of bloat!

I slowly lose more fat weight with time: As I mentioned, I now weigh 135 pounds and wish I weighed more. If I became ill with a prolonged illness, I might need these missing pounds to help me back to health.

What Researchers Say About Fructose

In 2020, Fryklund et al. commented that "Diets enriched in sucrose severely impair metabolic regulation and are associated with obesity, insulin resistance, and glucose intolerance" (https://pubmed.ncbi.nlm.nih.gov/32004930/).

In 2019, Pan noted that "Over the past few decades, epidemiological studies have demonstrated that high fructose intake is an etiological factor of metabolic syndrome" (https://pubmed.ncbi.nlm.nih.gov/29471102/).

[Metabolic syndrome includes high blood pressure, blood sugar, and blood lipids with increased fat around the waist.]

Caliceti, in 2017, observed that high fructose intake is a risk factor for high blood pressure, metabolic syndrome, heart disease, and probably for chronic kidney disease, diabetes, and cognitive decline [dementia].

(https://www.ncbi.nlm.nih.gov/pmc/articles/PMC5409734/).

Why I Reviewed Fructose

Excess fructose poisons us. Consuming fructose in excess predisposes the body to obesity, strokes, heart attacks, diabetes, dementia, and any condition to which we are genetically prone. These diseases strike many of us. If a little extra information helps you avoid illness, this review is well worthwhile. I want you to be healthy.

6

Refined Sugar: The Guide

Understanding Refined Sugar Is Understanding Dementia

Using what we know about fructose, we may find other harmful food chemicals. When we find them, we can avoid them or limit the amount we consume. This decreased intake should help us recover from many diet-caused diseases, including dementias like Alzheimer's, Parkinson's, and Lewy body diseases. Avoiding excess aging chemicals can heal the terrible destruction of our nervous system caused by our diet and give us the chance to live to old age with healthy bodies and young minds.

My migraine diet reversed my dementia and showed me that migraine headaches and dementia are similar. One similarity is that toxins (poisons) in our foods and beverages cause both conditions, and we can regard migraine headaches as a form of dementia. The headache pain in migraine headaches arises from damaged nerves like the nerve damage of Alzheimer's disease, with migraine's nerve damage directed at the nerves of the head and Alzheimer's disease directed at the brain's nerves. Indeed, nerve damage causes many conditions, and in each condition, the toxins in our foods and beverages may be part of the cause.

Join My Search for Causes

Use the information I have already developed about food toxins to see if foods are causing your distress. Also, join my search to find other worrisome food chemicals by looking for chemicals with characteristics of fructose. I find that avoiding excesses of the troubling chemicals —fructose, galactose, MSG, and citrus acids—prevents the severe dementia symptoms I suffered in the past. Perhaps, I have overlooked other chemicals that also damage our nervous systems, and you might find them. To help you recognize them, search for food chemicals with these characteristics of fructose:

- Fructose helps when consumed at tolerance.
- The body readily accepts fructose.
- Fructose tastes delicious.
- Fructose is a tiny molecule.
- Fructose dissolves readily in water.
- Fructose stimulates nerves.
- Domesticated crops contain fructose.
- Excessive amounts of fructose damage us.
- Excess fructose poisons the entire body.
- Drugs do not control fructose damage.

Fructose Helps When Consumed at Tolerance

We already discussed this. We tolerate and need fructose; our bodies will make fructose from glucose if fructose levels are too low. Fructose's ability to help the body store fat allows us to survive starvation. However, excess fructose causes disease, and avoiding consuming it in excess slows many diseases, as shown in the Mediterranean Diet's delay of dementia by limiting fructose consumption. Examples of this excess intake might include eating cherry pie with vanilla ice cream (sounds good to me) or drinking a sugar-sweetened carbonated beverage (sounds even better). Other food chemicals may share this characteristic; they poison us only when we consume them in larger quantities than we can handle.

https://www.ncbi.nlm.nih.gov/pmc/articles/PMC4496733/

This book does not discuss the illness called fructose intolerance. Your medical specialist treats this condition.

The Body Readily Accepts Fructose

The body accepts fructose and does not fight its passage into the body. This acceptance is not a good characteristic; it allows the excess intake to cause disease. In *Bioactive Food as Dietary Interventions for Diabetics* (2013), Jaffe describes what happens if the amount of fructose in sweet treats exceeds our tolerance. It floods us, overwhelming our digestive systems, inhibiting the liver's ability to digest fat, leading to obesity. In contrast, a high glucose level does not inhibit fat digestion; it helps the liver burn fat, raising the basal metabolic rate to burn off the excess fat.

Our bodies store much fat accumulated by excess fructose in the arteries, including those in the head and heart arteries, which predisposes us to strokes and heart attacks. Excess fructose also disrupts blood sugar, triglyceride (fat), and insulin levels. In addition, nerve cells survive poorly in this chaotic environment. Therefore, acceptance by the body is not always a good characteristic.

https://tinyurl.com/y5heqze6

Fructose Tastes Great

Absolutely!! Sweet treats taste great! What else needs to be said? But unfortunately, the sweetness attracts us, and we become addicted to this sweetness.

Fructose Is a Tiny Molecule

The tiny size of fructose probably helps it enter the brain. It readily travels through the blood–brain barrier that refuses entrance to other threatening chemicals dissolved in the bloodstream. I will further discuss the blood-brain barrier later in this book.

Fructose Dissolves Readily in Water

Fructose dissolves readily in water. This water solubility allows the sugar to dissolve in the bloodstream and reach every part of our bodies. This solubility has some benefits: It helps lower the amount of fructose in our foods; when we boil these foods, some fructose dissolves in the boiling water and we can then discard it.

Fructose Stimulates Nerves

You taste the sweetness of sweet food or a beverage immediately when you bite into it or take your first drink; the sweetness of fructose is a potent nerve stimulus. This stimulus does not harm the nerves of taste that send this sensation of sweetness to the brain. However, after we swallow the sweet treat, fructose travels through the body, overstimulating different nerve cells for days. Which nerves are most affected? Your genetic blueprint determines which nerves are most susceptible to damage from this stimulus; years of overstimulation eventually destroy these nerves and cause diseases like dementia.

Domesticated Crops Contain Fructose

Nature put only small amounts of fructose into crops. Farmers kept choosing the sweetest tasting plants, and they developed in plants like sugar beets and sugar cane, increased fructose sugar levels. Food manufacturers collect and use the fructose from these plants to make sweet treats. Honey, dates, and sugar maple sap also have increased fructose.

Excessive Amounts of Fructose Damage Us

I repeat this point because it is so important. As youths, we react less than older people to the fructose that nature placed in foods. However, we lose much of our tolerance to fructose as we become older.

Excess Fructose Poisons the Entire Body

Because it dissolves in the bloodstream, fructose penetrates every part of the body. Many drugs are examples of this poisoning by excess; they relieve disease at treatment dosages but can poison the body at higher doses. Water and salt also serve as examples of chemicals necessary for life, found in our bodies, and poisonous in excess. Drinking too much water induces a dangerous electrolyte disturbance. Consuming too much salt encourages diseases, including heart attacks. Fructose in excess is a poison.

Drugs Do Not Control Fructose Damage

Despite the billions of dollars committed to finding drugs to combat Alzheimer's disease, no drugs have helped, and no future medicines are likely to help. Researchers have already tried many medications, often with great expectation that they would help. They all failed. One reason for this failure is that our bodies recognize fructose as usual and not threatening; therefore, they do not resist it. Medications would have great trouble removing a chemical that the body regards as normal.

There is another reason drugs will not control dementias. The dementias poison us, like the poisoning caused by pesticides, cleaning products, poisonous mushrooms, etc. To treat this poisoning, you would not hunt for a drug. Instead, you would stop eating it and throw it away, which is the proper treatment for poisoning.

Limiting intake is not the treatment for potent toxins like cyanide, arsenic, or strychnine. In areas naturally containing these toxins, total avoidance is the best way to prevent their damage. Treat the aging food chemicals like these other poisons, by elimination, except they do not need complete elimination; they are mild poisons, bringing damage after years of excessive use. Food preparers only need to reduce their concentration in foods to a tolerable level.

I do not believe anyone is trying to identify a drug to block the more deadly poisons; if they are, I do not think they will find this poison-chasing wonder drug. Thankfully, the aging chemicals are not as lethal as cyanide, arsenic, and strychnine. The aging chemicals act much, much slower; instead of killing quickly, they kill after years of eating meals where they are in excess.

Scientists should give up trying to find a drug to treat the toxins of the excess aging chemicals. As mentioned, this excess can be treated today, at a much less expense, at the dining table, by limiting the amount of troubling chemicals we consume to the amount we tolerate.

https://www.healthline.com/nutrition/why-is-fructose-bad-for-you

Researchers' Comments

The information in Scott Edward's Summer 2020 Harvard Neuroscience Institute Newsletter, *On the Brain*, fits well with my thoughts. He mentions that glucose is the primary source of energy for all our cells. He states that eating or drinking too much of the simple sugar, fructose, ages our cells, agreeing with my thoughts about fructose and why I call it one of the aging chemicals.

A study at the University of Montreal and Boston College linked excess sucrose consumption to memory and cognition difficulties (dementias). I suspect that fructose contributes more to these difficulties than glucose because of the problems I listed above.

Vera Novak, MD, PhD, an HMS associate professor of medicine at Beth Israel Deaconess Medical Center, believes that diabetes, one of the consequences of fructose excess, "… accelerates brain aging," which accelerates dementia.

I felt uncomfortable calling the destructive chemicals—fructose, galactose, MSG, and citrus acids—the aging chemicals. However, as you can see by the above examples, experts agree that these chemicals, consumed in excess, *do* age us. Further, we know that scientists use galactose, the sugar in milk, to age laboratory animals in aging studies. For me, I have aged enough and do not want more!

What better name for these troubling chemicals than the aging chemicals?

https://diabetestalk.net/popular/sugar-and-your-brain-is-alzheimers-disease-actually-type-3-diabetes

Identifying Troubling Food Chemicals

Experts in developing and using healthy diets seem unaware of many threatening food chemicals that cause diseases. Unfortunately, these chemicals reside in our diet. Not all food chemicals cause distress; many fit the characteristics we discussed in this chapter but cause no harm. However, to preserve our minds and lives, we must be aware of the dangerous ones and limit or avoid eating and drinking them.

I know these troublesome chemicals target my nervous system, and I avoid or limit the foods and beverages containing them. Although I do not believe I have identified all threatening chemicals, avoiding or restricting fructose, MSG, galactose, and citrus chemicals reversed my dementia and obesity, which are great results.

I wish that everybody injured by these chemicals would change their diets, but I know that I cannot force anybody into this change. I can only hope that learning about my case helps those with dementia or who care for the afflicted understand dementia and use caution in what they eat and drink. And maybe they will find other threatening chemicals or invent better ways to remove them from our foods and beverages. That would be so helpful.

7

Monosodium Glutamate (MSG), Aspartic Acid, Low Calorie Sweeteners (LCS), and Gluten

Fructose Guides Us

Fructose shows us the characteristics of harmful food chemicals. This chapter will apply these characteristics to the amino acid, glutamic acid, a prominent amino acid in our diet and very dangerous.

Glutamic acid shares fructose characteristics, including being a life-sustaining chemical, helpful at tolerance, and accepted readily by the body. It is a tiny molecule, tastes excellent, and farmers grow crops with excesses of it. It strongly stimulates nerves and, in excessive amounts, damages these nerves. Drugs cannot control the whole-body poisoning of excess glutamic acid.

In *Escape From Dementia*, I discussed monosodium glutamate, also called MSG, the water-soluble form of glutamic acid. I separated MSG from low-calorie sweeteners and gluten because both form a large part of our modern diet. This book combines them into the same chapter to show that they are related because each contains glutamic acid.

Nature uses amino acids like glutamic acid to build proteins. It also uses glutamic acid and a sister amino acid, aspartic acid, to stimulate nerves; they are both neuro stimulants. Aspartic acid does not give foods a great taste, so farmers never chose aspartic acid-enriched foods to plant. In contrast, they developed many foods containing increased amounts of glutamic acid to make food taste delicious.

How Glutamic and Aspartic Acid Affect Nerves

Our nervous system enables us to perform many actions by sending nerve impulses along a highway of nerves, often beginning in the brain and continuing through succeeding nerves until it stimulates the desired activity. This nerve-stimulating process is like electric impulses traveling through a series of extension cords until these impulses light a lamp or start a motor. Like extension cords, nerves are covered with an insulating cover to prevent the stimulation from leaking away or short-circuiting other nerves. A covering called the myelin sheath serves these functions, insulating the part of each nerve—the axon—that touches other nerves. But how does the impulse pass from one nerve to another if the axon is insulated?

The answer: When a nerve impulse needs to pass from one insulated nerve to stimulate the next nerve, glutamic acid jumps across the space that separates the nerves, stimulating the next nerve. This space that glutamic acid crosses is called the synapse, and its function is to help the impulse from the stimulated nerve reach the next nerve needing stimulation. Without the synapse containing the nerve-stimulating glutamic acid, we could not act. We could not even live. Like the other aging food chemicals, MSG serves a vital need, allowing us to run, jump, chew, breathe, swallow, point and perform all the different actions that keep us alive.

Glutamic Acid in Our Diet

The glutamic acid that helps build proteins becomes locked into the protein. If it escapes this protein prison, this free glutamic acid, plus the glutamic acid from foods digested but not locked into protein, dissolves in the bloodstream. This oversupply of MSG travels throughout the body, overstimulating nerves.

Food manufacturers incorporate a lot of MSG in foods because it gives foods like fish, beef, and pork robust flavor, umami, improving the taste of the natural and manufactured foods sold in grocery stores. You find it on many food labels listed as a "flavoring" in processed food. In fact, I believe it is the chemical in food that is most responsible for the "processed" label.

MSG powerfully stimulates nerves. Just think of how quickly you taste the delicious flavor it promotes in the steak you eat; only one bite of the steak sends powerful stimulation to the brain's taste center. That's a potent nerve stimulator! A partial list of food products containing MSG is:

- Fast foods and commercially prepared meals
- Seasonings and condiments
- Instant noodle products

- Processed meats
- Chips, snacks, and soups

Add to this list fermented foods such as cheese and yogurt, which release MSG from protein in their preparation, and you can see that many foods contain MSG. The Food and Drug Administration classifies MSG as "GRAS" or **G**enerally **R**ecognized **A**s **S**afe.

Excitotoxicity

But is MSG safe? In "Glutamate as a Neurotransmitter in the Healthy Brain," Zhou notes that "Glutamate is the most abundant free amino acid in the brain … has excitatory effects on nerve cells, and it can excite cells to their death in a process now referred to as 'excitotoxicity'".

https://www.ncbi.nlm.nih.gov/pmc/articles/PMC4133642/).

Wikipedia defines excitotoxicity as the process by which excessive activation of the excitatory neurotransmitter glutamate (glutamic acid) damages and kills nerves. This excitotoxic molecule may be instrumental in stroke, traumatic brain injury, and neurodegenerative diseases of the central nervous system such as multiple sclerosis, amyotrophic lateral sclerosis (Lou Gehrig's disease), fibromyalgia, Parkinson's, Alzheimer's and Huntington's diseases, and others. That's a long list of common, terrible illnesses caused by MSG excitotoxicity! Other common conditions caused by neurons exposed to too much MSG are hypoglycemia and status epilepticus.

https://en.wikipedia.org/wiki/Excitotoxicity

MSG: A Slow-Acting Deadly Poison

The above statements worry me and convince me that excessive MSG is not safe. It can ultimately kill the sufferer. Consider this information:

"…most abundant free amino acid in the brain"

"…excitatory effects on nerve cells"

"excite cells to their death in a process now referred to as excitotoxicity"

The statements I quote above are unequivocal. Overuse of one of the tastiest flavoring agents in our diet, MSG, causes the debilitating diseases listed above. I believe that MSG is not safe when taken in excess; it should be used cautiously or not at all. Patients suffering from any disease should heed these cautions.

Too Much MSG

I stress that the amount of MSG in the diet determines how much danger it poses. There is no harm in eating small amounts. As with fructose, the mouth eliminates the MSG by swallowing it, so even large quantities of MSG-flavored food cause the mouth no injury. However, after swallowing, MSG floods the body, injuring nerves of the brain and body, especially the nerves weakened by defective or malfunctioning genes. I restate this point because it is essential: Only the mouth can avoid damage by passing on this nerve-stimulating amino acid; nerves in other body parts suffer damage. As MSG remains in the body for several days after a meal, it overstimulates nerves for several days.

When I consume excess MSG (believe me, only by mistake), I experience nights of poor sleep and days of not-quite-right thinking. For me and others with severe dementia, the sleep disturbance and thinking impairment caused by this over-stimulation last for one to three days, depending on how often I ingest it and how much I ingest. Higher quantities and more extended use prolong and worsen both sleep and thinking.

Unfortunately, many of us eat MSG-flavored foods daily for fifty, sixty, or more years—meaning this excess consumption continues for years. It continues until it deteriorates nerve-supplied organs of sight, hearing, balance, thinking, and other nerve-dependent activities. Damage can also occur suddenly; this neuro stimulant concentration increases in the stroke area and nerves die.

Once afflicted people end excess consumption, they gain a good chance of reversing these crippling conditions. And they start traveling the road to improved health.

https://pubmed.ncbi.nlm.nih.gov/20337054/

Aspartic Acid and Low-Calorie Sweeteners (LCS)

As I mentioned, aspartic acid, sister amino acid to glutamic acid, does not bother us because it lacks the great taste of glutamic acid. It is little used other than as part of a dietary sweetener with names like NutraSweet and Equal. I discourage using this sweetener.

In my opinion, LCS have one major failing. They are potent nerve stimulators, so powerful that only a tiny amount brings a pronounced sensation. The damage may involve those nerves that activate our hearing, seeing, walking, talking, thinking, and planning, seriously impairing these actions. These nerves keep us alive. I do not advise LCS use, especially in those severely afflicted with a disease or family history of these infirmities.

Gluten

We eat a lot of gluten in foods made from wheat, rye, spelt, and barley. Many vegetables contain gluten, but the gluten that concerns us most is present in wheat, barley, and rye. The status of oat's gluten content is uncertain. Wheat gluten holds together bread or cookies. Thirty percent of gluten (much of the protein in wheat) is the dangerous amino acid, glutamic acid.

Healthline lists the following as gluten-containing:

- wheat
- barley
- rye
- triticale
- farina
- spelt
- kamut
- wheat berries
- farro
- couscous

https://www.healthline.com/nutrition/gluten-food-list

People sensitive to gluten, and many believe they are sensitive, should watch out for this MSG sensitivity. When they suspect they react to a food or beverage, I have learned to respect their judgment: They are often correct. Indeed, gluten sensitivity can even cause ill-defined symptoms such as abdominal pain, bloating, diarrhea, constipation, "foggy brain," rash, or headache.

Processed Foods That Often Contain Gluten

- Beer, ale, porter, stout
- Bread
- Bulgur wheat
- Cakes and pies
- Candies
- Cereals
- Communion wafers
- Cookies and crackers
- Croutons
- French fries
- Gravies
- Imitation meat or seafood
- Malt, malt flavoring, other malt products
- Matzo
- Pasta
- Hot dogs and processed lunchmeats
- Salad dressings
- Sauces, including soy sauce
- Seasoned rice mixes
- Seasoned snack foods, potato chips
- Self-basting poultry
- Soups, bouillon, or soup mixes
- Vegetables in sauce

https://tinyurl.com/y9yfjwvs

Celiac Disease

Celiac disease is an autoimmune disease caused by wheat gluten that damages the lining of the intestine. Do not use this book to guide celiac disease treatment. Follow the directions of your medical care team.

Summary

Glutamic acid, in the form of MSG, is dangerous, destructive, and ages us. It causes many diseases through excitotoxicity. I urge you to learn more about this food chemical. Would you please try to avoid foods with excess MSG?

8

Citrus Acids

This chapter contains facts and speculation about the problems these acids cause. They worsen many diseases, including dementia, and you should know about them.

The Energy Hog

The brain is an energy hog. Although a small part of the body's weight, it uses much more than a small amount of the body's energy. This energy reaches the brain through a rich supply of blood vessels that bring much of our food energy to the billions of nerve cells and trillions of the connections uniting these nerves. All these nerves and connections require vast amounts of energy from our diet to perform their functions. A chemical cycle called the citric acid cycle is a series of chemical reactions used by all oxygen-breathing organisms to release energy from the sugar glucose. Although many diet experts regard these acids as safe, I believe citrus acids we consume are unsafe when we consume more than we can handle. Then they exhibit the dangers found in excess fructose and MSG.

Possible Reasons That Citrus Acids Are So Dangerous

Like fructose and MSG, citrus acids are life-sustaining chemicals that the body absorbs readily, needs absolutely, and enjoys immensely. They are tiny molecules, and each strongly stimulates nerves. Many fruits and vegetables grown for our consumption have excesses of these chemicals. I believe these excess acids damage nerves and cause whole body poisoning that no drug will control.

The excess citrus in our diet may disrupt the energy we harvest from our foods; the citric acid or Krebs cycle is an energy production process. When the cycle is overwhelmed, it causes or worsens many diseases, including dementias such as Alzheimer's disease. So, let's look further into these citrus acids.

A Review

The citrus acids include citric, malic, fumaric, and succinic acids from citrus fruits and tartaric acid from grapes and wine. They bring a refreshing citrus taste to foods and beverages and taste delicious. However, the following information suggests they also cause significant harm.

Eczema and Cold Sores

Two children taught me that these acids cause many, if not most, cases of eczema (atopic dermatitis). This rash is a chronic inflammatory skin condition affecting children (15%–20%) and adults (2%–5%).

https://www.ncbi.nlm.nih.gov/pmc/articles/PMC8010850/

As many as 35 million Americans suffer from this itchy rash. I treated many patients with this rash; reducing or eliminating citrus from their diets gave them tremendous relief. My readers who suffer this annoying and often unsightly rash should find comfort with this treatment.

Cold sores are another discomfort aggravated by the citrus acids. These sores arise from nerves that control the face, mouth, and lips and keep the skin healthy. However, these nerves are susceptible to a chronic infection by the herpes virus, which causes cold sores. These sores flare periodically, perhaps because another virus infection activates the herpes virus slumbering in the facial nerves. When activated, the facial nerves lose control of the facial skin, and a minor inflamed swelling called a cold sore appears, usually on the lips or in the mouth.

These sores affect a significant number of U.S. adults. I occasionally suffer these cold sores and find that consuming citrus acids changes my sores from minor, hard-to-notice swellings of the lips or mouth into angry-looking red splotches easily seen from a distance. Avoiding citrus when the cold sores appear prevents this rash from spreading.

The Grape Experience

I had a teaching experience while eating grapes. After several weeks of eating and enjoying grapes, the roof of my mouth swelled, most likely from the tartaric acid of the grapes damaging the virus-infected nerves that control the roof of my mouth. After I stopped eating grapes, the mouth swelling lasted for several weeks and then resolved, the top of my mouth returning to normal. Needless to say, I now avoid grapes.

Citrus Acids and the Brain

My experience with lip and mouth swelling makes me fear the acid's effect on the brain. Many of us harbor latent (inactive, sleeping) viral infections of the brain. Suppose another virus infection, like the common cold, activates this quiet viral infection.

https://askabiologist.asu.edu/plosable/sleeping-viruses

In that case, the brain infection may change from a sleepy condition to a red, swollen, and nerve-cell-killing brain infection when we eat citrus fruits or drink a glass of fluids flavored with one of the citrus acids. We would not feel the brain infection; we would be unaware that our acid treat is killing our brains' nerve cells. I worry about virus infections with the herpesvirus 6 virus and other viruses with the assistance of citrus acids causing other neurologic disorders.

Experts suspect viruses participate in neurodegenerative diseases like Alzheimer's, Parkinson's, and multiple sclerosis. This damage to the brain's virus-infected nerves may be a significant cause of the brain deterioration that accompanies these diseases, with the citrus acids worsening the injury.

Do not feed your loved one citrus juice to help control a viral cold or treat disease.

https://www.pnas.org/content/108/33/13734

Citrus Acids, Inclusion Bodies, and Brain Injury

If you suspect that I believe that fructose, galactose, MSG, and citrus acids are poisonous if consumed over tolerance, you are right. And, if you think we consume lots of these harmful chemicals because they taste so good, you are again right. Who would eat or drink citrus if they suspect it damages the brain? They who imbibe citrus—and our society—may be paying highly for this excellent taste.

Adding to Your Worries With a Suspicion: Inclusion Bodies

My suspicion involves the balls of protein called inclusion bodies found in the brains in dementia. We do not know how or why these bodies form, but I have a possible explanation. Amino acids link together to make proteins, much like a child connects one play block to another to build a house. Now imagine that some of the amino acids in a string of amino acids attract each other: imagine amino acid 22 attracting amino acid 45, and amino acid 16 attracting amino acid 56. These amino acids seek each other out, bond together like one magnet bonds to another, and the protein strings bend with these attractions, forming protein balls. Amino acids that repel each other further stabilize the protein balls, and the balls bend to accommodate this repelling.

This attraction and repelling of the amino acids in the protein curl the protein ball into a helpful form, the sequence of amino acids in the string determining their shape and function. They may look disorganized, but they are not; their shapes enable them to perform specific tasks. For example, some protein balls may split sugar, handle waste products of metabolism, or control the herpes virus. The controlled virus finds itself in shackles; it cannot attack the brain.

When Inclusion Bodies Form

The inclusion bodies identify the type of dementia. For example, the National Institutes of Health notes that balls of damaged proteins, called tau and beta-amyloid proteins, appear as inclusion bodies in the brains of Alzheimer's patients. Other inclusion bodies contain a protein, alpha-synuclein, identifying Lewy body dementia, and many cases of Parkinson's disease.

These protein inclusion bodies damage proteins and neurons around them. Researchers seek to discover the forces that turn beneficial proteins into the damaged Lewy bodies of Parkinson's disease and the plaques and tangles of Alzheimer's disease. We do not know why or how these inclusion bodies form, but I see a possible reason.

The acid of the citrus acids may cause these proteins to deform. Proteins are sensitive to the surrounding acid/base conditions, the acid denaturing many proteins, twisting and clumping them together. The citrus acids absorbed into the body from acidic foods and beverages may encourage these destructive processes; much of this acid goes into the bloodstream that washes the brain. Repeated brain flooding with acid from potatoes, tomatoes, apples, berries, grapes, and other fruits plus wine, candy, fruit juice, carbonated drinks, and other fruity treats makes proteins unravel. Then, when the acid disappears, they return to their previous form. This unraveling and reforming can denature proteins, including proteins of the brain's, turning them into destructive protein balls.

Damaging Protein Inclusion Bodies

Is this acid damage likely? After all, citrus acids are weak. Could the proteins that become unraveled be sensitive to these acids' action? It's possible. The acids that might deform the protein are weak, suggesting that they do not have the power to deform protein and form inclusion balls. However, the forces that hold the proteins together are also weak, including hydrogen, disulfide, hydrophobic, and Van der Waals forces. These weak connections may be susceptible to mild acid changes, making the brain protein they regulate vulnerable to the citrus acidity from our foods and beverages.

If this destructive process continues over many years—from childhood to advanced ages—it could denature protein and form inclusion bodies. In addition, it takes days for this excess acid from one meal or sweet treat to exit the body, so a citrus candy, a glass of orange juice, or a tasty citrus fruit can affect the body for days, magnifying the destructive potency of the mild acids. Thus, the inclusion bodies could develop from our diet's citric acid.

How Inclusion Bodies Cause Damage

How do inclusion bodies harm nerves? To see how this may happen, picture proteins as strings of amino acids (they *are* strings of amino acids). As I already mentioned, they do not stay in one long, straight line but bend into balls, with some amino acids attracting other amino acids and others repelling other amino acids. Perhaps these balls split sucrose into the two simpler sugars, glucose and fructose, so that we can absorb them into our bodies, or they destroy body toxins so the body can eliminate them. Or they battle the virus infections that sleep in our nerves. If the string loses its shape, it loses its power to split sugar, handle waste products of metabolism or, even worse, lose control of the herpes virus.

How Inclusion Bodies Injure the Brain

How does this group of damaged inclusion bodies injure the brain? Tau amyloid accumulates inside the brain's nerve cells; beta-amyloid accumulates outside these cells. The damaged protein plaques slowly increase in size and destructive power. The opening and closing of the protein balls with acid-base changes fuse many of them into dangerous unorganized jumbles.

Strings of separated amino acids now stick out of these inclusion bodies in all directions. These strings attach to other amino acids, including those in protein molecules wandering nearby, molecules innocently tumbling through the bloodstream. These unanchored strings may lock onto the amino acids in these nearby protein molecules, tearing them apart, rendering them useless and dangerous. Dangerous because these once-intact molecules are now damaged and can grab amino acids from nearby undamaged molecules. They can even cling to and damage the covering of the nerve cell itself, the cell membrane.

Protein balls must unravel and reform in company with other damaged brain proteins. In that case, in returning to their proper form, they may tangle together like a joyous family reunion with everyone hugging each other in one big group. These disrupted molecules may so severely damage the cell that it cannot eliminate the damaged protein, and the nerve cell dies. This whole process is a cause of dementia.

Beware of Citrus Acids

I feel so sorry for the people who must suffer from the itchiness of eczema, the disfigurement of large and persistent cold sores, and the dementias' progressive brain damage. These horrors do not need to happen. Not if we truly understand the poisons in our diet and take measures to lighten their impact. I believe that consuming excess amounts of citrus acids contributes to these horrors. I made it my goal to keep publicizing this possible acid-disease link until the medical profession acknowledges that the danger is valid or convincingly repudiates the concept. That has not yet happened. I do not know if diet specialists even consider the possibility that these acids are dangerous.

My Research on Citrus Acids

Please don't assume that this lack of knowledge is my fault. I wrote about citrus acids in an article titled "Atopic Dermatitis Associated with Citric and Malic Acid Intolerance" in the September 1979 Issue of *Minnesota Medicine*. Nobody paid any attention to my writing! I was so disappointed. I had to accept that the medical profession could not yet accept this information. Now, with the public knowing about the dangers of refined sugar, people may finally be willing to hear about other troubling food chemicals, including the acids' risks. If so, we can acknowledge that citrus acids should be consumed cautiously in dementia and other diet-caused diseases or not at all.

Hundreds of my patients with cold sores and eczema improved by avoiding citrus acids. I have avoided the citrus acids in my successful emergence from dementia. I do not doubt that citrus acids are toxic when we consume more than we tolerate and that poor tolerance is common. I would consider my life successful if others with dementia, including the dementias with Lewy bodies, Alzheimer's, and Parkinson's diseases, would avoid excess citrus.

The Citric Acid Cycle, Cori Cycle, and Glucose-Alanine Cycle

I mentioned that the brain is an energy hog. This energy reaches the brain through a rich supply of blood vessels that feed the billions of nerve cells and trillions of connections between nerves: These cells need energy from foods to function. The citric acid cycle releases this energy by degrading glucose. Then, other processes like the Cori and the glucose-alanine cycles restore the glucose, allowing it to go back into the citric acid cycle and produce more energy.

Energy production demands complicated chemical reactions, and it also requires discarding waste products or converting them back into valuable energy. This energy-producing process is impossible without a well-functioning citric acid cycle. The question arises: How do we know that flooding our bodies with citric acid does not disrupt this cycle? Unfortunately, we do not know. The nerve damage that citrus acids cause in eczema and cold sores tells me it is unsafe and damages the brain's nerves. We should limit citrus acids as we limit the other chemicals that age us.

Summary

The reason I write, and the reason I worry, is summed up in this description of Alzheimer's dementia by the Alzheimer's Association in "2020 Alzheimer's Disease Facts and Figures":

"Symptoms occur because nerve cells (neurons) in parts of the brain involved in thinking, learning, and memory (cognitive function) have been damaged or destroyed. As the disease progresses, neurons in other parts of the brain are damaged or destroyed. Eventually, nerve cells in parts of the brain that enable a person to carry out basic bodily functions, such as walking and swallowing, are affected. As a result, individuals become bedridden and require around the clock care. Alzheimer's disease is ultimately fatal."

https://tinyurl.com/y5almrel

I worry that citrus acids in excess are part of the reason dementias like Alzheimer's and multiple other diseases plague us and our society. The afflicted need not die from these conditions. Instead, if they change their diets, they gain a great chance to live a longer, healthier, and happier life.

9

Galactose

Like glucose and fructose, galactose is a simple sugar. I paid little attention to it until I read a diet study that brought galactose to my attention. It described how scientists in their aging studies use galactose to rapidly age the laboratory animals they study. An impressive number of studies use galactose to age laboratory animals because it accelerates aging by using a chemical pathway that our bodies use to make us older.

Oops! Another Simple Sugar to Worry About

Galactose shares many of the characteristics of fructose, MSG, and citrus acids. It is tiny, with only six carbon atoms. We need it to survive, so our immune systems recognize it as usual, do not attack it, but accept it and use it. If the levels of galactose drop below the average level, we can change glucose to galactose. It tastes better than glucose, encouraging farmers to plant crops "improved" by its taste. When we eat and drink more galactose than we tolerate, it ages us, probably because of its effects on nerves. I found no evidence that drugs prevent or reverse the nerve damage caused by galactose.

Neuroinflammation and Neurodegeneration With Galactose

The term neuroinflammation signifies the inflammation in nerves that leads to nerve degeneration. Britannica defines *inflammation* as a defense mechanism that evolved in higher organisms to protect them from infection and injury. It localizes and eliminates troubling chemicals and removes damaged tissue components so that the body can heal. Merriam-Webster defines *degeneration* as the deterioration of a tissue or an organ whose function diminishes or its structure degenerates. So, nerve inflammation leads to nerve degeneration.

Although dementias caused by nerve inflammation and degeneration are the focus of my books, many other common diseases also involve inflammation and degeneration. For example, inflammation and degeneration attend bacterial and viral infections, strokes, depression, hypertension, diabetes, dementia, and other conditions.

Neuroinflammation

Neuroinflammation has good aspects: Mild nerve inflammation helps repair damage to the brain, an excellent healing repair. More severe or persistent nerve inflammation does the opposite; it kills nerves. Consuming toxins daily in our meals makes neuroinflammation chronic, especially if between-meal snacks also contain galactose

https://en.wikipedia.org/wiki/Neuroinflammation

Neurodegeneration

Neurodegeneration affects the brain and spinal cord nerves, characterizing Alzheimer's, Parkinson's, and other diseases. Over five million Americans have Alzheimer's disease, and one million have Parkinson's disease. Multiple sclerosis is another neurodegenerative disorder affecting one million people. Amyotrophic lateral sclerosis (ALS or Lou Gehrig's disease) troubles thirty thousand people, and Huntington's disease forty thousand. These numbers are enormous. They overwhelm our health care system. Society pays a lot of money to treat neurodegenerative disorders.

https://en.wikipedia.org/wiki/Neurodegeneration

I do not mention this costliness as a plea to refuse these sufferers the treatment they need and deserve. Instead, I plead that the afflicted help treat themselves by reducing their intake of the troubling chemicals that age them. These chemicals—including galactose—aggravate diseases, afflicting many who might avoid or limit nerve deterioration by consuming less of this simple sugar.

Finding Galactose

Milk Products Containing Galactose

- Butter, butterfat
- Buttermilk
- Casein, calcium & sodium caseinate
- Cheese, cheese powder
- Cream, sour cream
- Fouche, fromage frais
- Ghee
- Hydrolyzed protein (from milk protein)
- Ice cream
- Lactose

- Margarine (containing whey or milk products)
- Milk, non-fat, skim or milk protein
- Milk solids, non-fat, skim milk solids
- Milk sugar, sugar of milk
- Skim milk powder
- Whey solids, whey syrup sweetener, hydrolyzed whey protein, whey powder
- Yogurt

Food Products Containing Galactose Not Made From Cow's Milk

- All animal milk (human breast milk, goats' milk)
- Lactose-free products (lactose-free milk, cream, yogurt, and custard)
- Chickpeas (bean flour, chickpea dahl, hummus, falafel)
- Legumes (dried peas, beans, lentils)
- Fermented soybean products (miso, tempeh, natto, soy sauce)
- Offal meat (liver, kidney, brains, pate)

http://www.agsn.org.au/food-and-diet
http://www.galactosemia.org/diet-resources

Foods Highest in Galactose and Not Derived from Milk

- basil
- beets
- celery
- cherries

- corn
- honey
- kiwi
- oats
- peas
- plum
- spinach

https://nutritiondata.self.com/foods-0000140000000
00000000-2.html

My Experience With Galactose

I wish I had more experience with galactose. I have experience with refined sugar, MSG, and citrus acids; they increase my patients' dementia and my own. But I have little experience with galactose. When I discovered how much damage it can cause, I was surprised. I was also surprised that researchers use galactose to age animals in their studies and that galactose fits well with all the food chemicals that accelerate aging. So, galactose has a well-earned place in the group of chemicals my diet avoids.

Do I believe that galactose belongs in the aging chemicals? Yes. I do!

https://tinyurl.com/yy36newl

Using This Information

How should you use the information I present? In the following chapters, I will discuss what you should do with this information.

One last comment: I do not know many people—beyond

their teen years—who want to speed up their aging. Instead, I am sure that, like me, they want to slow down, or even better, reverse aging. We can do this to some extent. Avoiding the chemical excesses that age us should help reverse aging: I feel much younger following my diet. I will continue to limit the aging chemicals because I want to continue to feel youthful.

10

The Trouble With Vegetables and Fruits

Toxins (poisons) in our diet come from two sources. We reviewed the first source, the aging chemicals including the amino acid, glutamic acid, the simple sugars fructose and galactose, and the citrus acid group.

As I mentioned in earlier chapters, and I will now repeat, although our bodies store and use the chemicals that age us and, although we need them to live, we suffer when we consume more of them than the amount we can digest and metabolize. These excesses are the prime causes of many diseases of the body and mind. For the young, consuming more of these chemicals than they tolerate temporarily dulls their thinking and planning. As we age, these excesses encourage more severe diseases, including obesity, strokes, heart attacks, and dementia. To combat these diseases, we must reduce our intake of these aging chemicals, and I showed you where they hide in our foods and beverages. Later I will tell you how I prepare my meals to reduce these excesses.

Poisons in Fruits and Vegetables

Now, we will examine other foods that also contain toxins—vegetables and fruits. Toxins in these foods are caused by:

- Contamination by microorganisms
- Natural toxins found in vegetables and fruits

Contamination by Microorganisms

Contamination by microorganisms hides in our vegetables and fruits. Microorganisms like campylobacter, salmonella, E. coli, and listeria release contaminating chemicals onto vegetables and fruits; we eat these toxins when we eat these foods. Our meats are also contaminated; we clean and freeze meat to slow this contamination and cook meat to destroy germs already in the meat.

Natural Toxins From Vegetables and Fruits

Vegetables and fruits also produce toxins to discourage predators like animals, birds, insects, and mold from eating them. Below is a list of plant-produced natural toxins and, for an example, a link exploring one, the lectins:

- Aquatic biotoxins
- Cyanogenic glycosides
- Furocoumarin
- Lectins
- Mycotoxins
- Solanines and chaconine
- Poisonous mushrooms

- Pyrrolizidine alkaloids

https://www.webmd.com/diet/foods-high-in-lectins#1-2
The World Health Organization cautions regarding natural toxins from fruits…:

- Do not think "natural" is necessarily safe.
- Discard bruised, damaged, discolored, and moldy foods.
- Discard food that loses its fresh taste or tastes unusual.
- Avoid possibly poisonous mushrooms and plants.

https://www.who.int/news-room/fact-sheets/detail/natural-toxins-in-food

Vegetables and Fruits Defend Themselves With Poisons

Vegetables and fruits are poisonous. To appreciate the toxicity of the chemicals produced by the plant, think of a garden of vegetables with beans, corn, lettuce, spinach, or any vegetable growing outdoors. We plant the seeds of these vegetables in soil with uncounted germs waiting to infect them and millions of insects that want to eat the seed. Despite this array of seed-killers, the seeds sprout, grow and mature into an adult food plant even though rain tries to make it moldy, and insects, birds, and animals would love to eat it. Plants survive these lethal threats because their poisons defend them from these plant predators.

Further, imagine apple, pear, walnut, and orange trees bearing their fruits. Why can't mold, insects, and animals dine on the fruits? Because tree-produced toxins protect the tree and its fruit.

Plant Poisons and the Blood–Brain Barrier

Plants are little chemical factories constantly making toxins to defend themselves. When Nature designed us, it knew that our nerve cells would be too delicate to survive exposure to the toxins our food plants produce. Plant poison threatens our entire nervous systems—central, autonomic, and intestinal. Did Nature design us to tolerate these poisons?

Nature designed all organisms needing plant food to survive the plants' toxins. We need this protection whether the plant is corn, cabbage, carrots, apples, oranges, or any vegetable or fruit. Many toxins attack the brain; Nature designed our brain and the brain of all creatures with central nervous systems—whether the systems are as simple as that in a jellyfish or as complicated as in humans—to tolerate these toxins. The protection is a barrier that shields the fragile brain nerve cells, *the blood–brain barrier*. It keeps our nerve cells alive and active despite the poisons we consume in our foods and beverages because the toxins in our foods and drinks would easily injure nerve cells in the brain.

The blood–brain barrier tightly coats the insides of the blood vessels that deliver energy to the brain. The barrier resists the entry of dangerous chemicals into the brain, shunting them away from the brain to the rest of the body that tolerates these poisons better. It is as capable a barrier as Nature can form, but it is not a perfect barrier: Nature does not make perfect barriers. As I mentioned, even in childhood, some toxins get through the barrier and enter the brain to lower the IQ.

With age, the barrier progressively fails, allowing more toxins to enter the brain, where they injure and ultimately destroy nerve cells. In addition to age, inflammation, smoking, and infections also degrade the barrier. Head injury and a flawed genetic blueprint increase this damage, allowing the trash-bag of toxins in foods to enter the brain and cause dementia.

https://en.wikipedia.org/wiki/Blood%E2%80%93brain_barrier

An Unsafe Diet

Please believe me; our diet is not safe. All our foods are poisonous. We eat them because we have no alternative; we need the energy that food provides. We can tolerate a limited amount of these numerous poisons but develop dementia if we eat more than we can metabolize. Since we dementia-prone people cannot repair the leaking blood–brain barrier, we must strive as we grow older to reduce our meals' content of poison to the amount we tolerate. We do this by avoiding foods and beverages with excess amounts of these poisons and preparing our meals with techniques that lower the remaining toxin in our foods. We can recover the thinking, planning, self-care, and independence that dementias steal if we do that.

As we delay the onset and then recover from these diseases, this diet provides an extra reward that I already mentioned and here repeat. It reduces the obesity that promotes conditions of body and mind like depression, anxiety, heart disease, diabetes, and strokes.

New Nerve Cells: Other Actors in a Deadly Drama

Immature nerve cells joining the brain keep it young and active, but only if they reach the brain while still alive! The food toxins poison these baby nerves before they reach the brain. Without the infusion of new nerve cells, the brain becomes shrunken, incapable, and old. We become old, demented, and die. The toxins in our modern diet orchestrate this catastrophe.

Although we should be concerned about the toxins in our food and beverages, we should realize that we can tolerate a certain amount of toxins without apparent harm. Keeping the amount of toxin-bearing foods in moderation lets me avoid worsening symptoms, and consuming these lower levels of toxins does not significantly increase my dementia.

Summarye

I reduced the amount of food poisons in my diet, allowing me to stop dementia's progress and recover from this disease. Others may be able to follow my diet and gain this same reward. To do this, they must reduce the poisons in their diets to an amount they tolerate; I know no other way to worm out of this disease's control. To evaluate how closely they should follow the diet, they need to recognize that our sensitivity to these poisons increases as we age. My sensitivity is now high: When I was young, my sensitivity was less, and as I aged, the sensitivity increased, increasing my need to avoid these poisons. Even though I became increasingly sensitive to foods, my increased avoidance slowed and reversed the march of my dementia. I know there are others like me able to follow my path to escaping this monster.

11

Further Information on Toxins

You may find it hard to believe that all the food we eat and the beverages we drink contain poison. I agree that this is hard to believe, but they do have poison.

I told you about the aging chemicals. I still find their ability to age us surprising. Fructose, galactose, MSG, and citrus acids join plant toxins in causing aging by aiding neuroinflammation that progresses to neurodegeneration. These two processes age us and destroy our nerves, and ultimately ourselves. Ferrucci expresses this far more scientifically: "Most older individuals develop inflammageing, a condition characterized by elevated levels of blood inflammatory markers that carry high susceptibility to chronic morbidity, disability, frailty, and premature death." I agree, and my diet lowers toxin consumption, decreases inflammation, retards aging, and has not yet killed me.

https://pubmed.ncbi.nlm.nih.gov/30065258/

Wikipedia's List of Poisonous Plants

On Wikipedia, I found a good source of information about poisonous plants. Wikipedia notes that many of the plants we eat have toxic parts or are toxic at certain stages of growth; we need to avoid these poisonous parts if we can avoid them and reduce their toxins if we can't avoid them. Some toxins poison only particular animals or certain people, such as infants, the aged, or those suffering from certain disease conditions. Other toxins poison all who consume them.

Onion, garlic, leek, and chive contain thiosulfate toxic to dogs, cats, and some types of livestock at high doses. Asparagus has poisonous berries, so growers harvest the asparagus before the berries fully form.

Most citrus fruits, including lemon, lime, and orange, contain oils and psoralen toxic to dogs, cats, and other animals (and, in excess, to us). Apple seeds contain small amounts of amygdalin; mango leaves, stems, and sap contain urushiol and poison ivy oil. You can find cautions about cassava and potato in the Wikipedia article. It is the same for nutmeg, rhubarb, lima, and kidney beans.

Cherry, peach, plum, almond, and apricot contain amygdalin in leaves and seeds. The stems, leaves, and unripe fruit of tomato, potato, and other nightshade family members contain solanine. Tomato has a small amount of the poison, tomatine.

Wikipedia, in "List of Poisonous Plants," lists other poisonous plants. There are many! It helps us realize that every plant must produce toxins to save itself from predators. I vividly remember a picture of husked corn with many worms crawling over the corn kernels. The corn plant did not have the poison necessary to repel these worms—an excellent example of the need for protective toxins required to grow a good cob of corn.

https://en.wikipedia.org/wiki/List_of_poisonous_plants

The Unknown Poisons in Foods

I believe that we have not identified all the poisons in our diet. I continually search for other toxins by checking my weight daily and using weight gain as a sign that I am eating or drinking a chemical that causes bloating; losing weight tells me that I stopped eating or drinking this toxin. Increased bloating means a food or beverage is damaging my nervous system. Then I figure out which food or beverage most likely is involved and avoid it or limit it. As I react promptly to correct the cause of the weight gain, I notice no permanent injury. I particularly worry about butter and olive oil; I dropped five pounds when I stopped cooking with olive oil. Butter may also harbor toxins, and I use it to help drive out toxins.

Poison on the Label

The label with many ingredients is a sign of trouble. I may be uncharitable and wrong, but I am hesitant to purchase it if the labeling uses more than one line. If the ingredients occupy more than two lines, I read no further; I leave the preparation on the grocer's shelf.

You may not expect to encounter toxins from plants in the various meats, fish, and fowl you eat, or the beef, pork, chicken, turkey, hen, salmon, and trout you enjoy. If food manufacturers use flavoring or seasoning in processed food or beverages, the flavoring or seasoning likely contains excess aging chemicals. Look for flavoring or seasoning listed on the food label and avoid buying it.

Even if the animal or fish is not seasoned or flavored, toxic chemicals may still lurk there, ready to damage nerve cells.

The foods recently eaten by the fish, animals, or fowl are still present in their bodies. Grass, hay, or other feed consumed by the cattle, pig, chicken, or turkey will still be in the animal's flesh for days after they eat it when you place the cooked food on your dining table. Fish seem to be less of a problem in dementia, perhaps because they dine on foods from the waters they inhabit, and we are not as sensitive to these foods as we are to grazing or carnivorous food. I suspect that birds are less threatening than plant-eating animals because their diet is different. Also, they may eliminate damaging chemicals from their bodies more rapidly than other animals and thus have lower toxin levels when cooked.

I know from my own experience that the foods we eat and the liquids we drink take at least three days before they leave the body. Therefore, unless the animals we use for food starve for three days before preparation, which I doubt, the poisons will still be in the animals when we eat them. In severe dementia, we need to eliminate these toxins as much as possible.

Water-Soluble Versus Lipid-Soluble Toxic Chemicals

This need for eliminating toxins brings up the following topic: water solubility versus fat solubility. In our food preparation, we need to reduce two types of toxin molecules—those toxins that dissolve in water (*water-soluble*) and those that dissolve in fat (*lipid (or fat) -soluble*). In cooking I boil the food in salt water to encourage any toxins that dissolve in this saltwater to leave the food, migrate into the water used in cooking so I can discard it.

I know that many toxins will dissolve only in a solution with fat. I already mentioned that I had used olive oil to cook my foods to drive off fat-soluble toxins; experts agree that olive oil is a healthy oil, and boiling olive oil in saltwater may dislodge some toxins from the food. When I read that some diets discourage the use of olive oil, I thought, *Whoa, am I making a mistake using olive oil?* To find the answer, I stopped using it and noticed weight loss within days. The weight loss answered my question: Olive oil carries its own toxin. I should have suspected this, because, like other food plants, olives need defensive poisons to deter predators.

Then I read about the wonders of butter and started using it. It worked wonderfully and gave an extra good taste to foods, so I added it to the saltwater boiling as I prepared meals. And I stopped using so much butter in my food preparation when I realized my memory was deteriorating. Within days, my memory started to limp back. It is now better than it was before I began to use butter. Now I use a small pad of butter to boil my food, hoping that this small amount will help dissolve lipid-soluble toxins, which I then dispose of when I discard the cooking solution. This limited use of butter does not worsen my dementia.

I tested my memory by picturing the home I left years ago. I remembered every floor of the house, the basement, the living floors, and the attic. I even remembered the home cupboards. My recall was good; I enjoyed recovering so much of my memory. If I had not changed my diet, I would not have remembered the house or other scenes that are sleeping in my memory. Further, I would have died already, killed by severe dementia. I *love* being in control of my memory and my life.

Review

I regret having to avoid healthful oils. However, I must do so to fight my dementia. I hope that this look at the toxins in the foods we eat and beverages we drink daily will help you better understand that we must fight diseases by lowering our consumption of these poisons. The dementia-afflicted should avoid cooking oils and butter other than the small amount that helps remove the lipid-soluble toxins in our foods.

12

The Value of the Books and Videos

I gave you much information about how the foods and beverages in our diet become poisonous and lead to many diseases when consumed in excess. How do you remember all this information?

Using Books and Videos

My series of videos on my website at drwewalsh.com tells you much about recovering from dementia. This book supplements this information and presents it to you in more detail. We learn by both the spoken and the written word, and the videos and books allow me to deliver information to you in both modalities. The time required to orally present information is much longer than the time necessary to read the information in a book; thus, books can be more detailed than videos and carry more data. Combined written and spoken presentations enable the book to supplement the videos and the videos to supplement the text.

The videos have advantages over the book; you can see me and judge the value of my information as I present it. Both books and videos have a place in your life.

Let's now further examine the value of the book. You may be experiencing symptoms caused by the aging chemicals and want to review where you encounter them in your diet. You can check this information in my *Retaining the Mind* series by paging through these books. Review your diet and then decide if you are avoiding these troubling chemicals. Are you reducing your intake of vegetables and fruit and preparing them for eating in a way that reduces their toxins? If you are not, you can avoid eating and drinking the foods and drinks you suspect are troubling you for a few days to a few months (yes, it can take months to recover your health). If you feel better, you can return to the diet that caused your symptoms to see if your symptoms worsen. If they do, you are right to be concerned about your diet.

The diet I suggest reverses my symptoms and may similarly relieve your symptoms. If you determine that these foods and beverages trouble you, continue to follow my diet.

Our Memories Can Fail

With time, our memories tend to dribble away. Few people can read a book or listen to an oral presentation and remember all the information they read or hear. Shortly after reading a book or attending a presentation, you will remember only some presented information. With a book, you can quickly return to the section you recall poorly and review the information. As time passes, more of the information I give you will fade from your memory: You may find the aging chemicals too many and the troubling foods and beverages more numerous for you to easily remember. Maybe, in a year, you will notice your symptoms increasing, possibly because you are returning to your previous diet without realizing it.

All these possible reasons for forgetting what I tell you can be counteracted by reading my books. They serve as your long-term memories when your short-term memory fades, and your memory will eventually fade. Keep my books nearby, close enough to reach out and remove them from the library shelf. They will quickly bring back the information you can use to help resist any disease.

Two Additional Advantages: Careful Wording and Sufficient Time

With a book, I can spend time presenting the information I want to give you. I revise each chapter many times, and then it passes the inspection of my editor.

Another advantage of the book is that I am under no time restriction on delivering this information to you. My oral presentation is limited to twenty minutes, one hour, or too infrequently, two hours. With time limits in an oral presentation, I must rush through the lecture and leave some of my message unspoken. This time limit does not happen in a book.

Two More Advantages

1) You need a lot of information to help you understand how I recovered from Alzheimer's dementia.
2) I enjoy writing.

13

Beginning My Diet

Two critical questions: At what age should you start the diet, and how closely should you follow it? Let's begin answering these questions by looking at the early years of life.

Providing Food for the Young

As we pass into our older years, the diseases caused by our diet become evident. As adults, we have, for years, consumed the aging chemicals. You would think that the young eating our modern diet for only a few years would not be affected. This thought is not correct; our diet also hurts the young.

A study by Mireia Adelantado-Renau and colleagues from Jaume 1 University in Castellon, Spain, tested the diet sensitivity of the young. They studied 269 adolescents, both boys and girls aged around fourteen years old. They divided these adolescents into two groups, one group following the Mediterranean diet and another consuming our modern diet. They found that adolescents with greater adherence to the Mediterranean diet scored higher in language, core subjects, grade point average, and verbal ability. (They also probably gained relief from the anxiety surrounding stressful events like tests; studies show that low-toxin diets like the

Mediterranean diet quiet anxiety.) Further, they found that this group gained better quality sleep and that sleep positively influenced academic performance. In other words, they slept better than the group eating our modern diet, the sound sleep contributing to their better test marks.

https://www.researchgate.net/publication/276358301_ Adherence_to_the_Mediterranean_diet_and_academic_ performance_in_youth_The_UPDOWN_study

Why did the improved test results correlate with more restful sleep? Consuming too much of the chemicals that age us makes sleep restless and not refreshing; restful sleep strengthens minds. My experience agrees with these results: If I eat and drink only the amount of aging chemicals that I tolerate, I sleep well and awake refreshed. If I sleep well, I think better, remember better, and react much better to stressful circumstances. Therefore, in this study and my experience, good health depends on adequate sleep; I use the quality of my sleep to judge how well I am controlling my dementia.

Diet, Cognition, and Age

This test of children, and other tests, show that these aging chemicals poison us at every age. The two-year-old and the sixty-year-old eating ice cream nestled on top of a cherry pie and drinking a refreshing citrus drink are swallowing a lot of poison. Poisons hurt all our systems, especially our nervous systems. The ten-year-old and the sixty-year-old eating MSG-flavored steaks are also eating poison. The main difference between the young and the aged is that the senior is more susceptible than the child to diet-caused diseases like strokes, heart attacks, dementia, and depression. The young shake off the illnesses that elders find difficult to leave behind. I suspect that damage to the blood–brain barrier accounts for the increased severity of dementia symptoms in the elderly. Young people have suffered either no injury or minor damage to the blood–brain barrier, and it is still intact. Perhaps, we will eventually learn to repair this barrier, allowing older people to respond to fructose, galactose, MSG, and citrus acids like youngsters. Then they can tolerate a more normal diet with its delicious but troubling foods.

Preparing the Young for Challenges

Although the young do not show the same degree of damage to thinking and acting that older people suffer, they are still affected by our diet's poisonous effects. These troubling chemicals lower the children's test results below what they would receive if they consumed less problem chemicals. If their ability should rate a "C" with a proper diet, perhaps they instead scored a "D+" with a toxin-containing diet. Maybe this lower test mark holds them back a grade. If they should have achieved an "A," perhaps they received a "B+" instead. Maybe they need the "A" to enter a prestigious school or a high-powered organization at school.

Children taking tests should be in the best cognitive state possible with low anxiety in critical testing situations. They should be thinking and acting better. They should not be under the influence of aging chemicals. These food chemicals' anxiety-producing and mind-dulling effects last about three days until the toxin exits the body. After this exit, with a low-toxin diet for the next three to fourteen days, immature nerve cells can replace the nerve cells damaged by our usual diet. The brain becomes restocked with young, healthy nerve cells able to store new information. The child can take the test with a more youthful brain, feeling less anxiety, and achieving a higher grade.

Give the Brain a Rest

With the above thoughts in mind, during the week or two before a test, change the diet to let the brain rest and heal with restful sleep that refreshes it. Reduce the troubling chemicals in the diet by avoiding the foods and beverages that contain excessive amounts of these disturbing chemicals. The children may complain vociferously but be firm, tell them that you love them, and only wish the best for them. Then, please cross your fingers and hope that with your dietary help, they get better marks. Maybe then they will gain entrance to the prestigious school or institution. Understand that their fellow students taking the same tests may know this secret of preparation and gain good marks by changing *their* diet. Do not let them get ahead of your child.

It is also possible that raising a child on a diet without our modern diet's high levels of troubling chemicals may result in the child gaining a higher IQ. I find this possibility intriguing.

Other Stressful Challenges

I do not mean that tests are the only stresses people need to prepare for by careful diet choice. As a young adult, choose your diet carefully when playing sports, engaging in high-tension social events, or applying for the first job or a higher status in your present job. A week or two without those delicious drinks, sweet treats, sauces, soups, and processed meat may pay huge dividends.

When I discuss dementia before an audience, the audience usually contains people of mixed ages. The young adults listen attentively, showing they are interested in learning more about a healthy diet. This group will nod yes as I speak; they are already aware of much that I discuss. Their close attention also indicates that they will consider following my advice.

As the children grow into young adults, their dementia symptoms should be only mild, and they need only change certain aspects of their diets. They may limit their consumption of sweet treats, processed meat, or carbonated beverages. Or other foods and drinks that contain excess troubling chemicals. This partial diet change may delay the onset of dementia for a significant time, maybe years.

Like the children I discussed, if these young adults desire to attend medical, dental, or veterinary school, a lower grade may prevent them from entering. Before the tests, for several weeks, they should be extra cautious in choosing their foods and beverages.

Before Stressful Times

I know that it would be better if everyone changed their diets to restrict troubling food chemicals. However, I believe that people at any age will avoid following a severely restricted diet unless they know that the diet helps them. As we have discussed, even slightly changing their diets in the years before these symptoms appear is valuable. It allows people destined for dementia to become familiar with partially following a healthy diet that delays diseases for years. They will find it easier to choose their foods and beverages in slow, more tolerated steps instead of having to radically change their diets as it becomes more evident that dementia is stealing their thoughts and memories.

My Diet Changes

Once my dementia symptoms appeared, they became very noticeable. My sleep deteriorated, my thoughts slowed, my conversation became difficult. And my memory turned sour. With these worrying symptoms, restricting the foods and beverages I enjoyed was difficult but necessary. Still, I found that the longer I denied myself these troubling chemicals, the more comfortable I was with choosing proper foods and drinks.

Until we know how to stop these diseases without a restricting diet, it remains the only way to reverse and escape many illnesses, including dementia.

I discussed easing into a healthy diet slowly in my first book in this *Retaining the Mind* series. When I advised patients to change their diets in my medical practice, I felt uncomfortable when they agreed to the change too readily. If they started compulsively following the diet, they would become bored and give it up. However, if they began the diet slowly, they would find it easier to learn to carefully choose their foods and increase their avoidance of dangerous foods as their symptoms worsened.

Preparing for Future Diet Restrictions: A Review

Experimenting should help people identify foods and beverages they must avoid as their dementia progresses. Once dementia starts, it probably will worsen unless they change what they eat and drink. Some food tolerable at forty years of age will become damaging at sixty or seventy years old. Suppose they continually experiment as they age and continue identifying and avoiding the foods and beverages that trouble them. In that case, they have an excellent chance to spend their later years in good health with an intact mind and memory, still driving a car and enjoying a fun life. And an extended life. What's wrong with living until 110 years of age in good health and with lots of other happy 110-year-old friends also following this diet.

Diet for Older Adults

People with dementia notice they are developing signs of this disease as they age, especially when using the same foods and beverages they used as youths. As it happened to me, in the early stages of dementia, they may not notice the onset of disordered thinking and memory. In my case, I was unaware of how much my mind had deteriorated until I stood up in front of an audience to introduce a speaker and found that I could not read the introduction I had prepared.

If the dementia-prone know the aging chemicals and how they destroy the brain, if they read my books, see my videos, or hear my presentation, they become aware of the cause of their deterioration and fight it by changing what they eat and drink.

It is never too late to experiment with food and ease into a dementia-controlling diet. The initial recovery from dementia may start only after some months of following my diet. If the diet I describe helps those with dementia, they should stick to it strictly, refusing the sweet treats, MSG-flavored steaks, age-inducing galactose, and refreshing, thirst-quenching citrus drinks. They can experiment with their diet, but only after they follow it long enough to determine if the diet reverses their dementia.

To determine if the diet helps, look for decreased weight, better sleep, and more inclusive memory as you follow it. If these symptoms improve, the diet works. There may be a time when the brain damage is too severe to gain much from the diet. Whether a diet change would help these severely damaged people is a discussion best held with clergy, friends, and family. I believe that my diet may rescue even the most severely demented.

Let me again mention that anyone contemplating diet change should only do so after their medical caregiver's evaluation and treatment.

A Summary and Preaching Moment

My dietary approach helps me and may help you or your loved one. Do not complain about the delicious foods and beverages you must avoid if you find these foods increase your dementia. You are trying to gain an unbelievable reward—fighting and defeating a disease trying to steal your mind and life. It takes real effort to reverse severe illness. I began fighting it before my loved ones forced me to stop driving my car or move into a memory care unit. If I had not taken measures to restrict these aging chemicals, I would have become too severely brain-damaged to reverse the deadly dementias, and I would have been housed in a memory unit without the ability to drive a car. I also would have died years ago. Unchecked dementia is a deadly disease.

I often wonder if the patients in a memory unit followed my diet, how many would return home to an independent life after a year. My guess is that many would regain much of their mental alertness and be able to go home.

I hope my diet gives you some ideas about controlling dementia. Then, despite dementia trying to kill you, you will be able to drive a car to Florida to help a friend move instead of lying in a bed on a locked ward waiting for someone to come to clean you up after a poor night of sleep. This image of myself in the messy bed haunts me; I hate this image. It keeps me loyal to the diet.

There is no doubt in my mind that dementia starts in childhood. The aging chemicals dull the youngster's competence sufficiently to measure on IQ tests. The significant difference between children and adults is not that children cannot suffer dementia but that they can emerge from mental dulling much quicker than adults. I do not advocate a strict elimination diet for the young. Still, I believe it is advantageous to cautiously begin teaching them about the diet at an early age, especially if there is a family history of dementia. Do not scare them or deny them the delight of tasting these delicious foods and welcoming beverages. Just let them know that they should be cautious about them and keep their portions small or avoid them when they must be at their best.

14

More Characteristics of the Aging Chemicals

Review: Fructose as our Guide

I discussed the characteristics of the aging chemicals when I discussed how fructose can guide us as we search for other threatening substances. Below are the factors I pointed out:

- Fructose helps at tolerance.
- The body readily accepts fructose.
- Fructose tastes great.
- It is a tiny molecule.
- It dissolves readily in water.
- Fructose stimulates nerves.
- Domesticated crops contain fructose.
- Excessive amounts damage us.
- Excess fructose poisons all the body.
- Drugs do not control fructose damage

In discussing MSG, galactose, and citrus acids, I indicated that they shared characteristics of fructose. Like fructose, these chemicals are poisonous when we take them in excess. They taste great, are tiny, dissolve readily in the bloodstream water, and the body does not fight against them because they are part of the normal body. Farmed crops contain these chemicals. They cause harm by damaging the nerves they stimulate. These chemicals penetrate throughout the body, and with drugs we cannot prevent the brain deterioration they cause. Avoiding excessive amounts is the only treatment.

I pointed out how to recognize and avoid them. Now I will show you other characteristics of these chemicals to help you better understand them and enlist your help to identify other troubling substances in our foods and beverages that I have not found.

Other Characteristics of Troubling Chemicals

- Aging chemicals damage all nerves.
- They operate together.
- The chemicals penetrate the blood–brain barrier.
- Our genes determine our susceptibility to disease.
- Aging chemicals and genes cause infirmities of the aged
- The aging chemicals age the brain.
- Excess aging chemicals and plant toxins harm all ages

Aging Chemicals Damage All Nerves

What parts of our body do the dementias most damage? They mainly damage our nervous systems. They induce difficulty thinking, planning, conversation, and self-care. Because of this nerve damage, the brain's nerve cells die, the brain shrinks, and we die.

The nervous system consists of three separate systems, the central, autonomic, and enteric nervous systems. The *central nervous system* directs our voluntary activities. If we run from danger, point our finger, or hop into bed, the brain sends the appropriate nerve activation impulses through the proper nerves to the right muscles, allowing us to run, point or hop. The central nervous system controls every voluntary motion.

The *autonomic nervous system* controls the internal organs that we do not consciously direct, such as breathing, heartbeat, and digestive processes. It activates the blood vessels, liver, kidneys, bladder, genitals, lungs, pupils, heart, and the sweat, salivary, and digestive glands. That's a big job.

The *enteric nervous system* is a subdivision of the autonomic nervous system that governs the gastrointestinal tract. Embedded in the lining of our intestines, beginning in the esophagus, and extending down to the anus, it regulates the contractions that move food along the intestinal tract until we eliminate it. It also regulates the secretion of gastrointestinal hormones. If disease disables the autonomic nervous system, the enteric nervous system takes control of the intestines.

We need to watch for distress in these systems to alert us to any damage. Excessive consumption of the aging chemicals ultimately destroys all three of these systems, making life impossible. Avoiding or limiting the aging chemicals before they ruin our nervous systems gives us a great chance of recovering.

I mentioned that we do not need to altogether avoid aging chemicals produced by plants because they are only harmful if we consume them in excess. But we do need to prepare these plant foods in ways that reduce their toxins. Refined sugar is an exception to this advice; it addicts us by its great taste, and, as in treating addiction, it is best to avoid eating any refined sugar. I know I should avoid any refined sugar; a little bit makes me want big bits of sugar. When we reduce the other troubling chemicals in our diet to the amount we tolerate, they do not harm us.

They Operate Together

The aging chemicals, fructose, galactose, MSG, and citrus acids, cause more damage because they operate together. Add toxins from our vegetables and fruits to these chemicals, and the combination becomes deadly. Without this combined attack by plant toxins and excess aging chemicals, dementia would not exist. Unfortunately, our meals usually include both aging chemicals and plant toxins. For breakfast, it may be a sugar-sweetened cereal and sausage with MSG; our beverage might be orange juice with citrus. We may enjoy an MSG-flavored burger and bun with mashed potatoes and a glass of carbonated sweet citrus beverage for lunch. Perhaps we will select an MSG-flavored steak and lettuce with MSG and acid-heavy tomato dressing for the evening meal, ending with a treat of cake and ice cream with fructose and galactose. In one day, we consumed excesses of fructose, MSG, citrus acids, galactose, and plant toxins.

These chemicals subject us to the nerve overstimulation of MSG, the acid disruption of the citrus acids, the aging effect of galactose, and the increased blood sugar, blood lipid, insulin resistance, and obesity caused by fructose. Our diets also add the poisons from plants found in vegetables, fruits, and meat to these chemicals. All these chemicals acting together multiply their damaging effects for the next several days before the body eliminates them. That's right. These poisons operate for days!

Although they are mild poisons, our daily consumption of these troubling chemicals over forty to seventy years exhausts the body, ages it, and brings or worsens multiple diseases. This effect is like consuming small, non-lethal doses of cyanide, pesticides, or other poison daily for years. No wonder we suffer so many destructive diseases. How much better off we would be without heart attacks, strokes, depression, and other disorders of the mind and body.

These Chemicals Penetrate the Blood–Brain Barrier

The blood–brain barrier protects the brain from harmful substances carried by the bloodstream. This barrier is composed of a tightly packed layer of cells and two membranes that coat the insides of the arteries carrying blood through the brain. This barrier allows helpful chemicals to reach the brain and resists the passage of poisonous substances.

The brain needs helpful food chemicals like glucose. Vera Novak, MD, PhD, an HMS associate professor of medicine at Beth Israel Deaconess Medical Center, notes: "It [the brain] cannot be without it." The brain demands enormous energy from foods, using a significant portion of the energy derived from sugar.

https://www.verywellhealth.com/what-is-the-blood-brain-barrier-3980707

Because of its solubility, glucose cannot move through the blood–brain barrier without the help of an intestinal transport system allowing glucose to move from the bloodstream into the brain. Fructose can penetrate the blood–brain barrier without a transport mechanism, which adds to the damage it causes when consumed in excess.

Why is this information important? Because we are trying to understand the dementias. Does a breach of the blood–brain barrier cause dementia? Studies suggest that barrier damage in the brain allows the destruction caused by dementia. The work of Berislav Zloislav of the Keck School of Medicine at USC shows that the gene APOE4, present in 10%–15% of us, hastens the blood–brain barrier breakdown, increasing susceptibility to dementia. Other studies agree that nerve barrier failure harms the brain.

https://news.usc.edu/153475/usc-alzheimers-research-leaky-capillaries/

With age or damage reducing the protection from the barrier, the chemicals that age us can sneak by its blockage and into the brain. Dr. Alan Gaby, a nutritional medicine specialist, suggested that excess fructose overloads the body's ability to turn fructose into glucose. It ships the excess fructose to the liver, causing liver inflammation and turning excess fructose into the fat that causes obesity, leading to the blood vessel, kidney, and eye complications of diabetes, strokes, and heart attacks. Add dementias to this list, and you can see that excess fructose is ultra-dangerous. (Dr. Gaby states that fructose *ages* people.) Isn't this why we suffer dementia?

https://doctorgaby.com/about-dr-gaby/

Our Genes Determine Our Susceptibility to Disease
Some ninety-year-old people are physically and mentally competent, and some fifty-year-old people pass away from

dementia. There is little doubt that our genes determine who dies early and who lives longer. It would be great to carefully pick our mothers and fathers to get parents with good genes. Unfortunately, we can't.

Aging Chemicals and Genes Cause Debilities of The Aged

Susceptible people have dementia because of their diet. Some of us suffer minimally, and some severely. I belong to the severe group. If aging people choose their diet with care (and prepare their own foods), the myth will fade that age, and not dementia, causes difficulty in thinking and planning. The toxins in our foods and beverages cause the infirmities of the aged. Whenever I see an older person walking with a cane or walker or using a wheelchair, I wonder if this assistance is necessary. What if they follow my diet? Could that bring back their ability to walk unaided? How about the poor near-blind soul desperately trying to read a book or watch TV? Or the near-deaf trying to hear a loved melody? Or the sufferer from dementia's dulling of mind and body trying to drive a car or prepare a meal? Are the delicious but damaging foods and beverages so appealing to these unfortunate people that they will not change their diet? I pray that they will try changing their diets, allowing them to seek relief from their distress.

The Aging Chemicals Age the Brain

Without the aging caused by fructose, galactose, MSG, and citrus acids, would the elderly brain be as young as the brain in a teenager? That is a possibility: I will discuss it in the next chapter, Old Brain/New Brain.

Excess Aging Chemicals and Plant Toxins Harm All Ages
Although the aged are most susceptible to the harmful effects of the aging chemicals and plant toxins, the young are also vulnerable. I pointed out that children, teens, and young adults suffer mental dulling, not necessarily severe but perhaps critical in a situation where a slight improvement in grades could determine a more advantagcous education or a more desired occupation. I would appreciate further investigation of the diet's dulling effect on the young, an inquiry that I know is difficult to pursue. In the meantime, I believe a diet change before a stressful situation is worthwhile.

Knowledge Maintains a Healthy Life
If you know the causes of the dementias and other debilities arising from damaged nerves, and if you change your diet to avoid the excesses that cause disease, you significantly improve your chance of preventing or recovering from dementia. I hope my experience, knowledge, and diet will guide you. It continues to guide me to good health, clear thinking, and great happiness.

15

Killing Newborn Nerves

To Understand Dementia

To understand dementia, you should know why some people die at forty years of age because of severe brain damage and other people enjoy life with capable, fully functioning brains at ninety or more years of age. The difference between early death and prolonged survival involves the immature nerve cells of the brain. There are many causes of immature nerve cell death, and I will discuss a few that predispose to dementia.

You should know about the energy these cells need, a subject I briefly discussed. Life requires energy; without it, we are dead. Perhaps that is the definition of death, the loss of life's energy.

The body is a chemical factory that produces the energy we need for life. To make this energy, we absorb foods—sugar, proteins, and fats—and break down this food to extract energy. We then discard the broken-down foods into the cells or the fluid surrounding the cells. These broken pieces of food molecules are called free radicals or oxidants. Oxidants contain oxygen that readily reacts with other molecules in the cell and the cell membrane, damaging both cells and membranes. They act like little hyperactive dogs that bite the mail carrier's leg and won't let go. If these oxidants stay in the cell, they injure the cell and even kill it if their numbers overwhelm the cells' ability to dispose of them. If too many cells die, healthy tissue becomes diseased and inflamed, beginning or worsening many diseases, including dementia.

Protecting the Brain by Cleaning Up After Eating

Like the homeowner who sweeps up and disposes of broken glass, our bodies usually clear away these free radicals before they kill the cell. If the number of oxidants (or free radicals) is limited, there is no disease. However, if the diet leaves too many free radicals (too many pieces of broken glass), the cell is damaged and can die. Those of us who handle these excesses poorly develop dementia.

Fructose is one example of the oversupply of damaging free radicals. Sweeter than glucose, its taste encourages this excess consumption. Glucose is different. The body tolerates it in moderate excess because all body cells can metabolize glucose (break it down to gain energy). Not all cells can use fructose; the liver, the one organ that breaks down fructose, can handle only the small amount of fructose present in unsweetened foods. People with dementia poorly tolerate these excessive amounts of fructose, and any cell dealing with this excess becomes inflamed. Even the liver, the one organ able to metabolize it, becomes inflamed and develops fatty liver disease. Immature nerve cells are susceptible to the damages caused by excess fructose.

Adding the Impact of the Other Aging Chemicals

Fructose does not act alone. Recall that MSG is a *neuro*stimulator (stimulates nerve cells) and, in excess, a *neuro*toxin (nerve poison). We also saw that in excess, MSG is an excitotoxin, a bad actor. As we sip our soup or eat our steak with its delightful MSG flavoring, we add more MSG than we can use. Swallow a mouthful of a refreshing citrus drink, and we add another neurotoxin to the damaging brew we eat. And your stomach pleads with you, "Please, no more!"

Is it any wonder that our baby nerve cells die from these toxic chemicals?

Other Conditions Associated With Nerve Death

Depression

Depression may be associated with dementia. The Mediterranean diet helps relieve depression, strongly suggesting that removal of refined sugar from the diet of the depressed helps ease depression. My diet, also decreasing or eliminating the other aging chemicals, should also help alleviate depression. Whatever the reason for this association of fructose and depression, it suggests that my diet helps the depressed. It would be wonderful if reducing our use of the aging chemicals makes the days of the sad brighter.

https://www.dementia.org/depression-and-dementia

Infection

My research and experience suggest that infections cause or worsen dementia. A significant association exists between dementia and chronic infection with microorganisms, including spirochetes, viruses, and bacteria. In 2017, Judith Miklossy, MD, PhD, discussed this relationship in the *Journal of Alzheimer's Disease,* and her evidence points strongly to infection with microorganisms in dementia. She identifies infection as a cause of dementia and the death of immature nerve cells. Defeating chronic infection may help prevent the destruction of these immature nerve cells that keep the brain young.

I do not know how quickly immature nerves become infected, but I suspect it happens before the cell reaches the comparative safety of the brain. The inflammation that accompanies infection may be a cause of immature nerve cell death.

From the above information, infection, inflammation, and the aging food chemicals must severely injure these helpless immature cells. I understand that many of us house a sleeping virus infection in our brains. This quiet infection must make the host nerve cells susceptible to the aging chemicals' poisons, weakening the cells and killing immature nerve cells. As a result of Miklossy's work, we can add spirochetes to our concern about viral and bacterial brain infections.

https://tinyurl.com/yfa44dex

Head Trauma

Moderate to severe head traumas is a risk factor in Alzheimer's as well as other dementias. Professional athletes who suffer a brain injury serve as examples; Mohammed Ali was a well-known example. A study of 7000 US veterans of World War II revealed that those who sustained head injuries suffered twice the average risk of developing dementia. The worse the head trauma, the higher the risk.

I often wonder if the cases of dementia associated with head trauma are clues as to why dementia primarily strikes the aged. Most likely, repetitive concussions from falling on ice, slipping on a carpet, playing friendly football games, and other head trauma episodes earlier in life permanently injure the blood–brain barrier and the cumulative damages from these traumas make the brain susceptible to dementia. Or unnoticed strokes may leave a leaking blood–brain barrier. These traumas could let dangerous substances enter the brain.

Genetic Predisposition

Known genetic abnormalities cause a minority of cases of dementia. Laura Sanders provides a good illustration in "Outrunning Alzheimer's" in the February 2020 *Science News*. She notes that most people with Alzheimer's suffer a sporadic form of the disease with no genetic cause and describes a family where a mutation in a gene called presenilin 1 causes family Alzheimer's disease. Other gene mutations also cause dementia.

This lack of genetic links to most cases of dementia does not mean that troubling genes do not cause dementia. It probably means that many genes cause dementia, genes we have not yet identified. Our scientists strive to find them, and I believe they will be successful in their quest.

Repopulating the Brain With New Nerve Cells

The brain does recover from damage. In my experience, acute symptoms of dementia from any cause last three days before starting to subside. For instance, after eating or drinking excessive flavored food on Sunday, my symptoms, including bloating, continue until Wednesday and then considerably diminish by Thursday. That's when I notice a decrease in my bloating and a weight decrease. The symptoms last much longer if I continue my diet, cheating for more than a few days. Eating excess troubling chemicals for years—as we do—may require several months of following a low-toxin diet before the symptoms of dementia subside.

In my hundred-pound weight loss, it took several months to lose the first five pounds. So, people using my diet to lose weight must be patient. It took about five years to lose the first fifty pounds and then another five years to lose the next fifty-plus pounds. Avoiding all sweet treats (fructose) lost the first fifty pounds; reducing MSG and citrus intake helped me lose the remaining fifty-plus pounds. If I had lowered my intake of food and beverage calories, the weight loss could have occurred earlier. But I didn't. I ate as much as I wanted, which was a lot of food. Remember, after this significant weight loss, I lost five more pounds when I stopped using olive oil and began using only a small pad of butter for my cooking.

This delay in weight loss may arise because the body is moving fat around in the body to where it can be easily discarded. I suspected this fat movement when I noticed that I was not losing muscle and bone loss, just fat.

In 2015, I noticed how severely dementia affected my speech. I also had great difficulty remembering names, places, and other information. I could only speak slowly with interruptions as I searched for the words I wanted to say. My speech was halting. I had to carefully plot out the words I needed to say instead of just saying them spontaneously. I still have infrequent trouble recalling specific words, and sometimes my sleep is poor, but over these many years of following my diet, both speech and memory wonderfully improves.

Each day, each month, my memory improves further, and I marvel at what I can now remember. (I still make some goofy mistakes, but I have a good excuse now—my dementia!) This continued improvement indicates that my brain continues to repopulate with new, young nerve cells; my brain recovery keeps improving.

If You Follow My Path, Be Not Impatient

Please do not give up because it takes so long to lose weight, regather your memory, and talk without searching for the next word. A slow weight loss probably means that you are not losing muscle and bone. You are losing fat! Appreciate your every improvement. Use this appreciation to urge yourself to continue following my diet.

Another Resource

You may want to explore the death of nerve cells further. I compliment you and suggest you consult an article by Michael Fricker, PhD, of The University of Newcastle, Australia, titled "Neuronal Cell Death." He explores nerve cell death, including death due to glutamate excitotoxicity, loss of connected neurons, aggregated proteins and the unfolded protein response, oxidants, and inflammation. (I will discuss excitotoxicity soon.) He also comments on cell death in stroke and Alzheimer's disease. I have touched on all of these topics. His article may increase your appreciation for the danger involved in using the aging chemicals, including MSG.

Please be aware that this is a long article packed with helpful information. The number of references he cites gives you a hint about the length of the article—807.

His knowledge again raises the question: If we know so much about why nerve cells die, why am I the only doctor who knows how to reverse this simple disease? The treatment is simple!

https://www.ncbi.nlm.nih.gov/pmc/articles/PMC5966715/

Killing Immature Nerve Cells

Depression, infection, head trauma, genetic blueprint, aging chemicals—all five have possible, indeed probable, roles in causing the dementias. They act together or singly. With these and other symptoms, be sure to involve your medical caretaker in your treatment.

People with dementia have already killed many of their immature nerve cells. This killing need not happen and is reversible! We can change our diet to reduce the excess aging chemicals at our dining table. It worked for me, and I pray it helps many others.

Let me be very specific: Do not follow my diet without first reaching out to the medical resources available to you. Illness not connected to your diet and having nothing to do with dementia may be causing your symptoms. If you do not consult other resources, you may miss a cure. If they do not find another cause for your symptoms, it may be in your diet. Then, you can investigate. Try my diet and find out if it is involved.

16

Dementia Is Not the Only Disease

Retelling Stories

I told you that I suspect that our modern diet injures my friends. To briefly restate their stories: those with sight loss can no longer enjoy TV programs or read a book. If my eyesight deteriorates until I cannot read books or watch TV, I will cry. They brushed off my suggestion when I suggested that their foods and beverages may be destroying their sight.

Another friend's hearing is failing. When I spoke to him, he completely turned his body to bring the ear with some hearing close to me. I told you that he was so frustrated by his hearing loss that he left the chapel where we met before I could suggest he investigate the possibility that his diet was destroying his hearing.

I regret that my friends did not listen. There is a strong possibility that the poisons in our diet are destroying nerves associated with their sight and hearing. The same food toxins that damage our brain in Alzheimer's dementia may be wasting these nerves, they cause Alzheimer's type diseases of sight and hearing. If my thoughts are true, strictly following my diet for the next year has a significant chance to slow, stop or even repair these nerves. It may return these wonderful functions of sight and hearing.

How Our Diet Injures Us

You might think that your foods and beverages bring you only good health. That is partially true, but foods also bring danger. They cause conditions like strokes, myocardial infarctions, lung emboli, diabetes, depression, and dementia; they worsen or cause any of the illnesses that afflict us. That's right; they make any medical condition worse. They help cancers arise and spread, as seen in studies of the relationship between cancers and the Mediterranean Diet.

Food's danger arises because we are eating the same plant-produced toxins that protect plants from predators. It's as if we sprayed our foods and beverages with an insecticide. How would you feel if a friend invites you to a dinner where you notice her spraying your food and drink with insect poison? You wouldn't eat her food, although, at every meal, you eat foods with similar toxins.

Diseases Other Than Dementia Are Important

Other than the dementias, body, mind, and psyche diseases can ruin our joy in life. Suffering from these other diseases can be as uncomfortable and threatening as suffering from dementia. An illustration of these other diseases happened to another friend.

A Case of Pulmonary Embolism

My friend called me and told me he had been in the hospital where he received treatment for an episode of breathing difficulty with swelling of his calf muscle. Tests showed that a blood clot from a vein in his leg broke free from the blood vessel and traveled to his lungs to obstruct the lung's blood flow. The obstruction, a pulmonary embolism, made him breathless.

Does this pulmonary embolism arise from the diet? It probably does. Can it be prevented by changing his diet? It should. Excess fructose of refined sugar makes us fat, which could cause the embolism he experienced. Suppose he follows a diet limiting the amount of fructose he consumes. In that case, it should reduce the fat in his leg veins, preventing another embolism, and this fructose avoidance is probably his most important treatment. As this excess fat predisposes him to pulmonary embolism, we can think that his hospitalization is because of an Alzheimer's disease of the lungs without dementia. (The internists might complain about that thought.)

When I lost over a hundred pounds, I could see that much of my weight loss came from eliminating excess fat from my body, lessening my chance of suffering a pulmonary embolism. Embolism is a potent threat to me, having lost two brothers to sudden death.

Another Diet Benefit

Another benefit of this diet: Embolisms may happen without recognizable symptoms. With so many of our fellow citizens overweight, could unnoticed pulmonary embolism from fat-corrupted arteries cause the puzzling tendency of the elderly to suffer hidden strokes? Obese people must be susceptible to these strokes. If they lost their obesity, would they suffer embolisms that injure the blood–brain barrier and allow nerve-killing toxins to enter the brain? If they have a genetic weakness to a stroke, these embolisms possibly arise even in people with an average weight. If they come to me for advice, I would advise them to follow a diet that reduces this tendency to stroke and lets the brain repair itself.

Another Reason to Write

It helps me interrupt my work on this book and reflect on why I dedicated my life to helping those suffering from the diseases caused by the poisons in our modern diet. The following is an experience suffered by a dear friend that will tell you why I continue this mission.

Her Eyes Begged Me to Help Her

Her eyes begged me to help her, but I couldn't help her. Her eyes still haunt me. We were grade school classmates with the same birthdate, and for many years we renewed our friendship with a birthday date at lunch with our spouses. Then we fell out of touch. I tried several times to call her, but she did not return my calls until that morning. Her conversation confused me as she struggled to tell me that she suffered progressive mental deterioration, diagnosed as Lewy body dementia, and it was destroying her! I was so sad!

She knew I had recovered from Alzheimer's dementia by diet change, and she asked me if diet change would help her. I hurried over to her house with a copy of my book, and she met me at the door. Her dementia was apparent, her conversation almost unintelligible, and her eyes begged for help. I could see that she would gladly try anything that may help her, but I worried that, in her confusion, she would be incapable of following my book's instructions. So, I turned to her husband for help.

He would not respond to me. He sat fifteen feet away, watching TV, and would not look up from the TV. I suspect that his apparent desire that I leave his house arose from a combination of factors. He might have lost hope that she could recover from her evident mental deterioration; he may have heard from her doctors that they could not stop her decline; he might suspect that I was working on some scam. I wasn't.

Although she wanted my help in reversing her dementia, I could not stay in her house to prepare her meals. I recognized that I couldn't help her beyond giving her my book, hoping that she, a relative, or a friend would try its suggestions. My diet should reverse her evident mental deterioration; she could recover.

If the diet worked for her as it works for me, her dementia could be stopped and even reversed. I wished her the best and hoped someone could use my book's information to help her. Nobody did, and she passed away. I miss her friendship.

My Diet Can Help

I will return to the friends I mentioned. Would you bet that the diet is responsible for their sight, hearing, and thinking deterioration? It would be a good bet. The poisons in our diet could cause their distressing symptoms and changing the diet could reverse them. They had the opportunity to read my book; I wish they followed its suggestions.

I have dedicated my life to help sufferers escape the mental fog of dementia, but sometimes I find my efforts heartbreaking. Too little, too late, and not believed. Discouraging.

Why I Try

I feel like crying when I reflect on the unfortunate people who suffer from our modern diet. Their stories profoundly sadden me. These diseases, and other nerve-damage debilities, affect millions of people. Changing the diet can be done at home, continued if it helps, and stopped if it doesn't. A diet change is not overly expensive. It is far less costly than living in a memory unit. I believe that the chances are excellent that if they followed my diet, my friends and millions of others could recover their mental abilities sufficiently to make the change worthwhile. This thought keeps me on my mission. As long as I am able, I will continue.

17

Barrier Failure, Excitotoxicity and MSG

R ecent scientific studies shed light on dementia, especially on the role of MSG in dementia. I believe this is the proper time to look at these studies.

The First Study: Poison and the Gene

Ted Turlings, PhD, and his colleagues at the University of Neuchâtel in Switzerland reported in "Plant Gene Has Naturally Crossed into Insects – And Helps Them Feed" in *NewScientist*. The plant gene, BtPMaT1, has never previously been found in insects. The insect is the silverleaf whitefly, an aphid-like insect.

The gene serves a vital function. We discussed how plants generate toxins (poisons) to defend themselves from damage from animals, mold, and insects. BtPMaT1 may help plants store the toxins in a form that avoids poisoning the plant, poisoning only the animals, insects, and mildew that would destroy the plant. This plant gene transplanted into the whitefly must be allowing the insect to eat the poisonous plant.

What We Learn From This Study

This study adds to our knowledge of dementia by confirming what we already know: Plants make many poisons to defend themselves. The whiteflies avoiding poisoning by the plant toxin raises a question: We also know why we are eating vegetables containing toxins. The answer: Because we need to eat plants to feed ourselves. If we want to eat peas, beans, lettuce, broccoli, and other food plants, we must eat the toxins that protect the plants. Unfortunately, in certain predisposed people, eating these plant toxins causes dementia. However, without the poisons, we would not have any foods; all plants depend on toxins to keep themselves alive.

We also discussed how our bodies try to protect us from these plant poisons, by using the blood–brain barrier. It shields our most delicate organ, the nerve cells in our brains, from plant poisons. The barrier does not give us complete protection; even in our youth, Nature cannot provide an impenetrable shield. In people susceptible to dementia, protection deteriorates as we age, subjecting us to increased poisons in the foods that make their way through the barrier into our brains.

Many experiences make the blood–brain barrier fail, including trauma to the head and various brain infections.

In the study Neuronal Cell Death, you met many of these causes of cell destruction and dementia. The study below discusses gene failure and dementia.

https://tinyurl.com/yfvuhovw

Demyelinating Diseases and Dementia

This study was published in *Aging Cell* by Professor Arthur Butt at the University of Portsmouth and international colleagues and titled, "Myelin Loss Plays Key Role in Age-Related Brain Deterioration." The authors studied the brain's white matter where the axons reside and make connections to other nerves. We discussed how these axons act like electrical wires that connect all the different parts of our brains. Insulating coverings called myelin sheaths prevent axons from touching and short-circuiting other axons. The progressive loss of this insulating myelin characterizes the aging brain.

The myelin sheath needs to be continually replaced by stem cells that differentiate into cells called oligodendrocytes. These cells support and insulate axons in the central nervous system, including the brain and spinal cord. The Schwann cells in the peripheral nervous system serve the same function as the oligodendrocytes. (The peripheral nervous system includes the nerves that begin in the brain and spinal cord and extend to the rest of the body, including muscles and organs.)

Professor Butt's group found that the gene, GPR17, guides oligodendrocyte replacement, allowing immature cells to replace the older cells. Weakening of this gene reduces this protection, enabling progressive barrier damage that leads to increased brain destruction. With the loss of this protection, we think, plan, speak and act poorly. Eventually, we no longer live.

What We Learn From Myelin Loss

These studies help us understand diseases.

The myelin loss in the aging brain causes or worsens dementias like Alzheimer's, Parkinson's, and Lewy body diseases. Common autoimmune diseases like multiple sclerosis exhibit myelin loss. Other demyelinating conditions are palsies, migraine headaches, depression, and anxiety. Poorly restrained anger, various addictions, attention and cognitive deficits, and eating disorders also accompany myelin loss. As you can see, demyelinating diseases are many, millions of people suffer from them, and they can be devastating.

To discuss the dementias alone without mentioning these other demyelinating diseases makes us overlook the seriousness of blood–brain barrier deterioration and its consequences. It enables us to entertain a fallacy that dementia is the only disease promoted by demyelination. No—every disease is affected in a minor or major way.

https://neurosciencenews.com/myelin-loss-aging-neurodegeneration-18005/

https://tinyurl.com/yg8qyhsk

Excitotoxicity in Neurodegeneration and Demyelination

Excitotoxicity is the overstimulation that damages nerves, and neurodegeneration is the death of nerves. Glutamic acid, one of the aging chemicals, transmits more nerve impulses than any other nerve impulse transmitter in the central nervous system of all animals, including ours. It is a significant cause of the overstimulation of nerves. Two studies give us insight into this overstimulation of nerves by glutamic acid.

"The role of excitotoxicity in neurodegeneration" discusses the work of Elzbieta Salinska and colleagues of the Neurochemistry Department at Mossakowski Medical Research Centre, Polish Academy of Sciences.

https://pubmed.ncbi.nlm.nih.gov/16416396/

"Glutamate receptors, neurotoxicity, and neurodegeneration"

describes the studies of Anthony Lau, neurosurgeon and assistant professor, Donald and Barbara Zucker School of Medicine at Hofstra/Northwell.

https://pubmed.ncbi.nlm.nih.gov/20229265/

These studies examine how neuro-stimulants such as glutamic acid cause the death of nerve cells. Dr. Lau points out that glutamate excitotoxicity occurs in chronic neurodegenerative disorders such as amyotrophic lateral sclerosis, multiple sclerosis, Parkinson's disease, and others. These diseases are some of the conditions associated with blood–brain barrier damage.

He further points out that there are currently no treatments that provide significant protection to the damaged brain. Could some help come from lowering the amount of glutamic acid (MSG) in the diet? I think so. This reduction of MSG would be like placing less poison in our meals, and that should help.

Reviewing Glutamic Acid, MSG, and Gluten

The amino acid, glutamic acid, makes up about a third of wheat, rye, and barley protein (soy also has high levels). When you're eating food with high levels of gluten, you're eating a lot of glutamic acid. This amino acid is typically locked in protein, but digestion frees it; it becomes MSG, the water-soluble form of glutamic acid. Glutamic acid-containing foods produce high levels of MSG. In many people, excess MSG leads to hyperstimulation and neurotoxin damage to nerves.

Combine MSG with the poison from toxins the plant produces to protect itself from predators, and you have dangerous nerve stimulation.

This relationship between gluten and MSG means that people with dementia should follow a diet low in MSG and gluten. I follow a low-gluten diet. The Mayo Clinic discusses a gluten-free diet, pointing out that exposures to gluten are many. Surprisingly many:

- beer, ale, porter, stout (usually contain barley)
- bread
- bulgur wheat
- cakes and pies
- candies
- cereals
- communion wafers
- cookies and crackers
- croutons
- French fries
- gravies
- imitation meat or seafood
- malt, malt flavoring, and other malt products (barley)
- matzo
- pasta
- hot dogs and processed lunch meats
- salad dressings
- sauces, including soy sauce (wheat)
- seasoned rice mixes
- seasoned snack foods, such as potato and tortilla chips
- self-basting poultry
- soups, bouillon, or soup mixes
- vegetables in sauce

This sensitivity to MSG and plant toxins, not identifiable by testing, may explain why many people experience undiagnosable symptoms that may be wrongly considered psychological.

https://tinyurl.com/yyparot5

What Are We Eating?

You are aware of the great harm these demyelinating diseases cause millions of people. When I hear the terms "demyelinating" and "sickness," I think of all the poisons we eat and drink daily. I know they are significant causes of our diseases.

Hunting for some drugs that will work in poisoning wastes time and money; throwing away the poison is the treatment for poisoning. We throw it away by changing the diet, and diet change should be the first treatment. After all, isn't eating a vegetable or fruit with its plant poisons the same as eating a sub-lethal dose of any poison, including insect spray or strychnine. Your food contains toxins that repel and kill mold, insects, and animals; how do you know if they encourage disease in you, your child, spouse, neighbor, or friend? It would be worthwhile to think about what you or a loved one eat and drink.

18

Measuring Dementia

If you have dementia, you are now aware that you are in the clutches of a deadly disease. You need to know if you are sinking deeper into its mind-robbing coils or if you can escape from its rotten embrace. You want to live; your dementia wants you dead. To continue living, you must measure its progression frequently, best daily, and appropriately respond if you notice your grip on life slipping.

The Bathroom Scale

The best instrument to measure your success or failure in fighting this disease is the bathroom scale. You should weigh yourself daily and record the weight the scale indicates. If you weigh more than you should when starting the diet, your weight should decrease until you reach a weight that your body decides is proper for you. I already discussed the system that holds my weight at a healthy level, and you should have the same system. Be patient. When you start following my diet, it may take a long time for the fat control system to gain control of your weight. You can tell if you are following the appropriate diet if your weight begins to drop. When you reach your body's desired weight, the scale should stop decreasing; it should show the same weight and display it for years if you follow the diet with minimal cheating.

My weight decreased from 248 pounds to 140 pounds and has remained at this level until recently when I noticed that it was slowly sinking to 135 pounds while fat attached to my abdominal skin noticeably decreased.

It took over twenty years to lose more than one hundred pounds, and I feel comfortable at 135 pounds. It is the right weight for me.

Progressively Worsening Symptoms

Other symptoms tell you if you are winning or losing your battle to control dementia. Its primary targets are our nerves. Since the nerves manage all our body functions, nerve damage symptoms can arise in any part of your body, letting you know that dementia is active.

Many good examples arise from my experience with my diet. I had been cheating on my diet, taking a small amount daily of a solution containing about a teaspoon of honey. As you know, honey has sugar and must have a significant load of toxins to keep it from spoiling in the flower, the bee's body, and the hive. After two weeks of cheating, I noticed that I was developing symptoms of Parkinson's dementia. I noted troubling stiffness of my body as I walked, feeling stiff and off-balance, needing considerable effort to move my stiff legs forward. Further, I forgot the names of the people I know well. I was astounded that such a small amount of sugar could cause such significant symptoms.

A Little Poison Can Be Too Much Poison

I immediately stopped using this small amount of honey and resolved to be more cautious of the foods I put into my mouth. This experience taught me, and now teaches you, a good lesson: Cheating has consequences. It doesn't mean that you can't cheat, but it does warn you to be careful of how much cheating you do; stop cheating if you notice increasing symptoms of dementia and be sure to hurry back to my diet if you find that your symptoms increase. It also teaches me that even a tiny amount of sugar and plant toxins can cause significant deterioration.

Preserving Immature Nerve Cells

I now restate our definition of dementia. *Poisons, also called toxins, contaminate all our foods. The body shields our brains from these toxins, but in many people like me aging degrades this shield and makes us suffer from dementia. Reducing diet toxins can lead to recovery.*

You're aware that toxins damage nerves. Immature nerve cells keep the brain young and free from dementia, but they must reach the brain to refresh and renew it. If we kill these new cells by our diet, the brain shrinks; it becomes incompetent. Eventually, it no longer keeps us alive, and we pass away. To prevent this, we must do our best to keep the immature nerve cells alive so they can improve our thinking and memories. We need to carefully follow a low-toxin diet that does not kill the immature nerve cells our brains need to remain young and healthy.

To make sure we are not consuming excess toxins, we should frequently weigh ourselves. If the scale shows weight gain, determine the cause of this increase. Is it the diet? Are the toxins in vegetables and fruits responsible? Could it be the toxins in meat, maybe the steak sauce used to flavor it two days ago? How about that cherry pie with chocolate ice cream that tasted so delicious? Perhaps the scale reacts to the MSG in the salad you enjoy at the restaurant you frequent? Whatever is elevating the weight is also killing the baby nerve cells. This killing should be slowed or stopped before the brain absorbs too much damage.

19

The Brady Superbowl Diet

Tom Brady, the quarterback of the Tampa Bay Buccaneers, won his seventh Super Bowl in 2021. In winning the Super Bowl, he showed that a proper diet can work wonders.

Tom Brady's Diet

In preparing to write about Tom Brady's diet, I reviewed many articles and studies that discussed his diet. After reviewing over 100, I chose several. "Tom Brady Diet Review: Weight Loss, Meal Plan, and More" from *Healthline* impressed me, as did *Vox's* "Tom Brady's Diet Book Makes Some Strange Claims About Body Chemistry." The information on his diet was similar in the many articles, including the Healthline and Vox articles.

Tom Brady developed this diet and describes it in *The TB12 Method*, his book about diet. He further teaches the reader how to decrease injury risk and improve athletic performance, energy levels, and overall health. I believe his diet does what it claims, mainly because it fits so well with my diet.

It's lonely trying to persuade others that the diet I must

follow to control my dementia works. I cannot blame my listeners or readers who doubt me; after all, how many people will follow a diet that removes many delicious foods and beverages that they crave, a diet that other diet specialists do not promote. Tom Brady's winning ways may help me persuade these doubters that dementia is a diet-caused disease. His success may convince the dementia community that they or their loved ones suffer an illness that they can escape by changing their diets. I am delighted that his experience may help me spread this good news.

A Healthful Diet

Some years ago, I read a magazine article about Tom Brady's diet and, sad to say, I do not remember the magazine or the author who wrote it. I hunted for this article but gave up after checking over 150 articles. I do remember how I felt after reading his story; I was delighted. The article mentioned that Tom considered himself just an ordinary football player before following this diet. With the diet, he became extraordinary. This transformation from ordinary to exceptional may seem too much to believe, but it isn't. He stopped eating and drinking much of the toxin-containing foods and beverages in our modern American diet. With this decreased dietary poisoning, his body responded with clearer and quicker thinking and acting under stress (being chased by the opposing team is *very* stressful), faster recognition of the opposing team's defense, and a younger, more athletic body. This response is not surprising. It is expected. After all, if athletes daily eat sublethal but significant doses of poisons at one to three meals, they will not perform at the same level as athletes that eat lower, more tolerable levels of these poisons. He discussed this in an interview in the past.

https://en.wikipedia.org/wiki/List_of_poisonous_plants

Seven Superbowl wins firmly state that his diet is healthy. I believe that it also argues that my diet, a similar diet, is also healthful. I will discuss the diet changes in both diets that feature reduced toxins and could elevate an "ordinary" player into an extraordinary player.

The TB12/Walsh Diet

I know that I am claiming too much by adding the name of Tom Brady's diet, the TB12 Diet, to my diet, but I can dream, can't I? How could anybody—including myself—claim to have anything in common with this marvelous athlete? I might have one claim to fame: As he shows how to improve athletic ability, I show how to recover from dementia. Now, let me be serious and analyze his diet and compare it with mine. I will discuss:

- The TB12 and Walsh diets are healthy.
- Both diets resist aging.
- Our diets are appropriate for our ages.
- Both diets reward the follower.
- The diets are home-based medical care.
- They lower the cost of medical care.

The TB12 and Walsh Diets Are Healthy

The TB12 Diet is healthy. Anyone who can win the Superbowl as often as he has must be healthy. Not only did he play the quarterback position well, he was also chased all over the field by the opposing team of super athletes. To survive, he had to be healthy. If his diet is unhealthy, years of eating it will keep him off the field, especially at forty-three years of age. Like Tom, any athlete of any age in any sport will better compete by following his diet and recommendations found in TB12.

My diet is also healthy. In 2015, my dementia lowered my ability to talk and think, and I was on the path to death; without changing my diet, this disease would have killed me years ago. Not only did my diet rescue me from death, but it also allowed me to live, speak, and give hour-long discussions about dementia and my disease-fighting diet. It allows me to keep writing books, hoping they save other disease sufferers from becoming dependent on others for eating and dressing. It saved me from being placed in a memory unit and then hospice to await the final visit of this "always lethal" disease. For many people sensitive to foods, my diet is healthy. (Always remember to use my diet under the supervision of your medical caretakers.)

Both Diets Resist Aging

Once we pass the ages of thirty to forty, we become more interested in staying young. If I gave you a glass of milk and told you it would age you, you would refuse the milk and feel angry and insulted. You might refuse to talk to me again; that is an appropriate reaction because milk sugar, called lactose, contains an aging chemical, the simple sugar galactose. I already told you that scientists use galactose to age laboratory animals when they study aging. It works very well.

Olivia Tarantino of *Eat This, Not That* reported that Tom and former chef Allen Campbell developed his diet, and Tom still follows it. His diet avoids galactose, one of the four aging chemicals I already discussed. In a 2016 interview in the Boston Globe, Allen Campbell related that Tom does not use dairy products, including milk, cheese, and yogurt. Thus, his diet avoids the aging chemical galactose, thus avoiding the aging of this chemical.

He also avoids refined sugar. Refined sugar in excess is a toxin leading to several adverse conditions, including inflammation, obesity, diabetes, and metabolic syndrome (high blood sugar, high blood lipids, waist-level fat, and high blood pressure). Both my diet and Tom's diet discourage this excess.

His diet also discourages MSG, another of the aging chemicals. His avoidance of flour, soybean, mushrooms, cheese, and yogurt limits the glutamic acid that changes to MSG with digestion. However (a "however" hides in everything), his protein shakes probably contain glutamic acid, which turns into MSG with digestion. If they do, this high-MSG protein does not degrade his abilities and age him because he is young, and a diet that avoids only some of the food toxins may be enough to improve his athletic performance. I will return to this thought soon.

His diet further avoids the nightshade family with potatoes, pepper, and tomatoes because he believes these foods cause inflammation. I agree. Tomatoes contain appreciable quantities of citric, malic, and ascorbic acid. Lemons, limes, oranges, and grapefruits all contain significant citric and ascorbic acids, and apples contain higher levels of malic acid. I have already mentioned my concern that acid food may be causing the protein disruption that creates inclusion bodies that injure and help kill nerve cells. The presence of plant poisons augments this death threat.

I agree with his avoiding fruits and fruit juices, thus limiting fructose, citrus, and plant toxins.

He worries about food-caused *inflammation*; I worry about food-caused *aging* caused by inflammation. Our worries are the same; *inflammation* from food toxins causes *aging* and *aging* from food toxins causes *inflammation*.

I believe I gave you enough information to show significant similarities between Tom's TB12 Diet and my Diet.

https://pubmed.ncbi.nlm.nih.gov/22742651/

Our Diets Are Appropriate for Our Ages

Many people ignore my diet because they think it is too strict for them at their present age. Many are right. In my eighties with severe dementia, the diet that I need to follow must be rigorous. I can still cheat on it if I do not cheat too much or too long. If I do, I start sliding down the path to the swamp of confusion. I quickly return to following the diet more closely and recover well.

At his age, Tom Brady has more freedom than I do in his food choices. For example, he is unharmed by his high-MSG smoothies that would increase my dementia. Because of his Super Bowl wins, we know that the smoothies and other troubling foods and beverages are not troubling him. He might have the genetic makeup that makes him susceptible to dementia, and if so, when he reaches his fifties, sixties, and seventies, he might need to follow my diet for the severely afflicted. At present, he does not need to be more cautious than he is about his food.

How closely you need to follow the diet depends on your age and the severity of any symptoms. Is it harmful to follow it closely while your symptoms of dementia are mild? Not if you continue to follow a healthy diet. If you limit all the aging chemicals, you may prevent dementia. It is best to be aware of your family's heritable diseases to see if you are susceptible.

Both Diets Reward the Follower

I do not need to point out the rewards of following these diets. Tom wins Super Bowls. I write books and do not mess my bed at night. Yuck!

For us, those rewards are magnificent.

The Diets Are Home-Based Medical Care

Absolutely! You sit at home at your table and select healthful foods and prepare them in a way that lowers their toxin content.

They Lower the Cost of Medical Care

I understand that the average cost for a private room in a nursing home is about $300 per day or $100,000 per year. On average, the cost of memory care is above $5,000 per month for a private room, about $60,000 per year. Eating either Tom's or my diet at home is far less expensive. The numbers of people with dementia increase steadily and may reach a level that our society cannot pay. Why not try to treat yourself by following my diet? It may control dementia for years, maybe for a lifetime. There is a chance that my diet will not help you, but you lose your chance of recovery if it would help you and do not try it.

20

The Paleo, Keto, and Carnivore Diets

Many Healthy Diets

We looked at the Mediterranean, DASH, and Mayo Clinic diets in Chapter 3: "A Healthy Diet." I believe it appropriate to examine other diets and see how they contrast with my diet. I chose three that are popular, the Paleo, Keto, and Carnivore diets. I will start with the Paleo and Keto diets and end with the Carnivore Diet.

The Paleo Diet

"The focus of the Paleo Diet is not on finding the ideal macronutrient ratio but on eating the foods we evolved to eat and avoiding anything processed." Trevor Connor, MS

The Paleo Diet website describes the diet. Dr. Loren Cordain, a professor at Colorado State University, developed The Paleo Diet® through decades of research and with fellow scientists' help. The diet is primarily plant-based. It encourages eating natural foods derived from plants while discouraging processed foods.

Sugar

Megan Patiry discussed natural sugars. She suggests that sugar from natural sources, such as honey, is less troublesome than refined sugar. However, even raw sugar taken in excess can lead to illness, including obesity, diabetes, insulin resistance, and leptin resistance. (Leptin signals when the consumer has consumed enough food). She also pointed out that, before the advent of our year-round supply of refined sugar, our ancestors could obtain sugar only during times of the year when plants with excess sugar grow. Thus, there was no reason for Nature to give us ancillary means of handling sugar other than the liver, even in these more modern times.

Megan cautions us to use natural sugars sparingly. I agree because sugar is addicting. I suffered months of sugar withdrawal when I stopped eating sugar, so best not to eat it at all.

Fruits and Vegetables

Professor Cordain finds excellent value in fruits and vegetables. As we poorly tolerate our present diet, the Paleo diet attempts to return us to our ancestors' foods. He urges the consumption of fresh, raw fruit and vegetable juice. He is also concerned about our diet's content of sodium, potassium, calcium, and magnesium. I share that concern.

The Nightshades

Megan discussed the nightshade vegetables—white potatoes, peppers, and tomatoes. They contain "deadly nightshades" (belladonna). The foliage and berries are extremely poisonous when ingested. Nightshades also contain natural "pesticides," alkaloids, and lectins to defend against pests. Sensitive people may react to these nightshade chemicals with intestinal irritation and worsening of any underlying autoimmune issues, including multiple sclerosis, arthritis, allergic inflammation, pancreatitis, diabetes (and the dementias, my contribution to this list).

Trever Conner discussed wheat sensitivity and the paleo diet. Many people who do not have celiac disease suffer from wheat that causes intestinal symptoms such as diarrhea, bloating, fatigue, and irritable bowel syndrome. Many of my patients suffered the same symptoms from wheat. He states that wheat causes the breakdown of the gut barrier that protects the body from intestinal bacteria. This breakdown allows the vast horde of gut bacteria entrance into the body, activating the immune system and causing inflammation.

Foods to Eat or Avoid on Paleo Diet

Foods to *include* on the Paleo diet include leafy and root vegetables, fresh fruits, nuts and seeds, herbs, seafood, grass-fed meat, sweet potatoes, and free-range poultry and eggs. The diet encourages healthy oils, including olive, walnut, flaxseed, macadamia, avocado, and coconut. Desired beverages are water and herbal tea. Foods to *avoid* include dairy products including milk and yogurt, grains including oats, pasta, and cereal, and legumes including beans, soy, and peanuts. Also avoided are potatoes, processed foods, refined vegetable oils, and added salt (sodium) and sugar. Use sparingly: natural sweeteners like honey, molasses, or dates. Also, used sparingly: coffee, beer, wine, almond and coconut flour, or other baking replacements.

https://tinyurl.com/y9vph7qy

The Keto Diet

The ketogenic or "keto" diet is a low-carbohydrate, fat-rich diet that aims to help control diabetes and drug-resistant epilepsy in children. It benefits patients with obesity, cancer, diabetes, polycystic ovary syndrome, and Alzheimer's disease.

Familiar diets like the Atkins, Paleo, and South Beach diets are high-protein and moderate-fat diets. In contrast, the ketogenic diet is average in protein intake and exceptionally high in fat content.

For the energy of daily life, the brain uses much glucose energy. However, it can run out of its stored glucose so, during fasting, the body first uses the liver's store of glucose. Then, when the glucose is depleted, the insulin that regulates glucose decreases, and the body turns for energy to the liver that produces ketone bodies from fat. The ketone bodies, instead of glucose, provide the body's energy.

The deficiency of glucose may in some way provide a therapeutic effect. However, without glucose, obesity and the many diseases that obesity promotes give less trouble. Various ketogenic diets encourage different ratios of carbohydrates, protein, and fat; commonly, about 70%–80% daily fat calories, 5%–10% carbohydrate calories, and 10%–20% protein calories. These diets provide only moderate amounts of protein because overeating protein allows the protein to convert to glucose. Then, the newly developed glucose prevents the ketosis these diets seek. These diets offer just enough glucose and protein to preserve lean body mass while still allowing ketosis.

Foods and Beverages Allowed and Avoided on the Keto Diet

Many versions of ketogenic diets exist, but all ban carbohydrate-rich foods. Suggested and avoided food lists can vary between diets and even conflict with each other. Some diets avoid starches from refined and whole grains like bread, cereals, pasta, rice, and cookies. Other diets might also limit potatoes, corn, other starchy vegetables, and fruit juices. Still other diets avoid beans, legumes, and most fruits. Some Keto diets avoid foods high in saturated fat, such as fatty cuts of meat, processed meats, lard, and butter. Some avoid sources of unsaturated fats such as nuts, seeds, avocados, plant oils, and oily fish.

Because of this variation, it is best to read and follow the Keto diet suggested by your medical caretaker. Here are a few points to remember:

- Keto diets are high-fat diets.
- They somewhat limit fructose, galactose, MSG, and citrus acids.
- Some Keto diets restrict dairy because of high milk sugar content (galactose).
- Some avoid grains (MSG) and sugars (fructose).
- Some Keto diets limit fruit.
- Some avoid legumes.
- Alcohol is limited.

Potential Pitfalls of the Keto Diet

Continuing to follow a very high-fat diet is challenging. Possible symptoms of extreme carbohydrate restriction that may last days to weeks include hunger, fatigue, low mood, irritability, constipation, headaches, and brain "fog". Though these uncomfortable feelings may subside, staying satisfied with the limited variety of foods available on the keto diet and being restricted from otherwise enjoyable foods like a crunchy apple or sweet treat may present new challenges.

Some adverse side effects of a long-term ketogenic diet have been suggested, including increased risk of kidney stones, osteoporosis, and increased blood levels of uric acid (a risk factor for gout). Possible nutrient deficiencies may arise if the dieter avoids some of the recommended foods on the ketogenic diet. The dieter should include a daily variety of the allowed meats, fish, vegetables, fruits, nuts, and seeds to ensure adequate fiber intake. Also important is including B vitamins and minerals (iron, magnesium, zinc), nutrients typically found in foods like whole grains that the diet restricts. Because entire food groups are excluded, seek assistance from a registered dietitian and follow an acceptable keto diet that minimizes nutrient deficiencies.

The Carnivore Diet

The carnivore diet is just what the name implies, a diet that depends greatly or only on animals, fish, seafood, and fowl. It encourages any foods from organisms that fly, walk, or swim that you can eat morning, noon, and night. According to *Carnivorestyle*, the diet encourages the following:

- Red Meat: Pork, Beef, Lamb, and Game
- White Meat: Turkey, Chicken, Fish, and Seafood
- Organ Meat: Liver, Kidney, Bone Marrow, Heart

- Eggs: Chicken, Duck, and Goose Eggs
- Dairy: Butter, Cheese, and Cream

Troubles With the Carnivore Diet

My first problem with the diet is not a significant problem; I do not eat lamb, liver, kidney, and bone marrow. Maybe I should. Avoiding dairy may be wise because of its galactose content. Glutamic and aspartic amino acids are significant components of milk proteins, and milk protein makes cheese, so dairy products' content of MSG is high. The more fermented the cheese, the more the dairy protein separates into amino acids and sugars, including fructose. Glutamic and aspartic acids are the primary amino acids in milk protein, released from their prison in the protein when we consume milk protein. Once free, these amino acids become neurotoxins if released in amounts above our ability to handle them. Most of the older people who have dementia do not need galactose to age them further. Time will increase our ages all by itself, but we can stretch out this time if we avoid chemicals that age us.

Foods Avoided on the Carnivore Diet

All foods are avoided except meat and dairy while on a carnivore diet. Avoided are fruit, dairy, and vegetables. Also avoided are sauces and most seasonings plus highly processed meat and alcohol, including beer and wine.

Concerns From the Agency

The International Agency for Research on Cancer (IARC) of the World Health Organization (WHO) specializes in cancer, as its name suggests. In October 2015, twenty-two scientists from ten countries met at IARC in Lyon, France, to determine the danger of consuming red and processed meat. Red meat includes beef, pork, lamb, and goat. Processing indicates that the meat is preserved or flavored with chemicals; processing can be by salting, curing, fermenting, or smoking in making ham, bacon, sausage, and some deli meats.

Stacy Simon of the American Cancer Society reported that experts estimate that eating 50 grams of processed meat each day increased colorectal cancer by 18%, elevating the lifetime risk of this cancer from 5% to almost 6%. There was a possible increased risk of colorectal, pancreatic, and prostate cancer for unprocessed red meat.

Cancer Risk
Although this is a regrettable increase in the possibility of cancer, it is a small risk. The risk of dementia posed by the aging chemicals in processed meats must be more significant than the cancer risk for red meat. Processed meats like sausages frequently contain the aging chemicals to improve the taste, and it is wise to avoid these processed meats.

Risks found in the study may arise, not from the meats themselves but from eating the toxins in our modern diet found in processed meats because of its aging chemical content. As studies of the Mediterranean Diet show, avoiding refined sugar helps cancer treatment. Reducing the consumption of the other aging chemicals and the toxins in vegetables and fruit must have this same cancer-inhibiting effect. These aging chemicals poison the entire body, and eating and drinking them for years must significantly increase cancer's likelihood and make it more challenging to treat. It must also make any disease more formidable.

Why should unprocessed meats have an increased risk of cancer, not as significant as the risk associated with processed meat but still increased? The cook preparing the meat dish perhaps adds seasonings or flavoring, probably containing MSG and other harmful chemicals, to red meat to improve its taste. If so, the seasoning and flavoring added by the cook may cause this increased risk of cancer in unprocessed red meat and not the red meat itself.

https://carnivorestyle.com/carnivore-diet/food-list/

Remembering All the Good Food

In Chapter 3 and this chapter, I told you about many diets recognized as healthy, including the Mediterranean, DASH, Mayo Clinic, Paleo, Keto, and Carnivore diets. Now comes the hard part—remembering which foods each diet advocates. For instance, the *Mediterranean diet* emphasizes eating fruits, vegetables, whole grains, beans, nuts, legumes, olive oil, and flavorful herbs and spices. It encourages eating fish and seafood several times weekly; and poultry, eggs, cheese, and yogurt in moderation while reserving sweets and red meat for special occasions. The carnivore diet recommends red meat: pork, beef, lamb, and game; white meat: turkey, chicken, fish, and seafood; organ meat: liver, kidney, bone marrow, heart; eggs: chicken, duck, and goose eggs: dairy: butter, cheese, and cream. That is an enormous number of foods to remember. Let me confess; I can't remember all of them either.

Easier to Remember

Let's try something more manageable: *Remembering why we avoid foods and beverages.* It is easier for me to remember that we avoid foods to reduce our intake of aging chemicals and plant toxins. So, we alter our diets to reduce toxins.

All healthy diets help their followers. Some even slow the progression of dementia. However, to recover from dementia, we must reduce the toxins that our modern diet contains. Fortunately, completely eliminating them is not necessary, and it is impossible. Every processed food and beverage we eat and drink contain toxins, and without these foods, we would have nothing to eat. It is sufficient to just reduce the toxin content in our diets to give us good dementia relief. Besides, we require the aging chemicals fructose, galactose, MSG, and citrus; we could not live without them. Our need to reduce our fruit and vegetable toxins consumption sounds like a prescription for poor health, but I have reduced them for years and feel fine. Also, proponents of meat-rich diets do not seem to develop diseases easily.

Our Rewards

There are rewards for changing the diet. The diet reduces the power of our foods and beverages to damage our brains. You would expect that people who are daily fed toxic foods would find our modern diets have troubling power to weaken resistance to disease and cancer, and I showed you evidence it does have this power. Further, a significant life event can be more easily faced and successfully completed while reducing these toxins. Those who follow my diet can gain significant rewards.

21

Preparing for the Diet

Your Knowledge Has Progressed

Throughout this book, I told you about the relationship between dementia and our diet. I will restate some of the components of the relationship before discussing the diet necessary to control this condition. First, let me reassure you that dementias are simple diseases where poisons, also called toxins, from our foods and beverages, seep through an increasingly incompetent brain barrier to destroy brain cells. This disease only attacks people whose genetic blueprint allows the attack.

- The dementias include Alzheimer's, Parkinson's, and Lewy body diseases.
- Alzheimer's and Parkinson's diseases affect me.
- The toxins (poisons) in our foods and beverages cause dementia.
- These toxins are chemicals normal to our bodies.
- They poison us when we consume more than we can handle.
- They also age us when we consume them in excess.
- Plants need toxins to defend themselves from predators

- All plants, including food plants, produce these toxins.
- We consume aging chemicals and plant toxins daily.
- Animals, fish, and fowl contain these toxins from eating plants.
- We eat these toxins as we eat the flesh of these plant predators.
- The cells most susceptible to these toxins are the nerve cells.
- After dining, the toxins stay in our bodies for three to four days.
- The blood–brain barrier shields our brains from most of these toxins.
- With age, the barrier deteriorates and we suffer from dementia.
- Careful food choice and preparation reverses dementia.

My Diet Reverses Many Diseases

A Quick Review

Our diet causes many diseases we already identified. In dementia, the site of the brain damage determines each dementia. Please understand that my diet can help relieve any disease condition, even such different conditions as depression and cancer. We can fight these diseases by reducing our intake of toxins which also protects the immature nerves that refresh our brains and keep them young.

Even if your condition is not dementia, your body and mind will suffer if you eat more toxins than your body tolerates as we see in studies of children following the Mediterranean Diet.

Home Self-Treatment

Changing the diet is a treatment that people can do at home. With this diet, the stroke survivor might walk with better balance and confidence. Or it could help the heart attack patient by removing some of the fat remaining in the heart's arteries threatening further heart damage. The diet may allow the brain damaged by dementia to recover its alertness. For me, my diet suppressed my dementia and returned much mental alertness; it may extend this help to others suffering similar brain damage.

These thoughts travel through my mind when I see people using walkers and canes as they recover from strokes. I want to tell them to change their diets to stop killing the immature nerve cells trying to reach their brains and repopulate the stroke-damaged areas. However, I do not have the right to interfere in their treatment unless they ask me. I wish they would ask me. I could give them valuable suggestions about allowing the brain-damaged areas to recover.

You have permitted me to give you advice about treatment by reading this book. I am so pleased.

Determining the Severity of Your Dementia

Before deciding how closely to follow my diet, you should assess the severity of your dementia. Many dementia symptoms arise from damage to the nerves in the central, autonomic, and gastrointestinal nervous systems control all body processes. To see if your symptoms flow from toxin-damaged nerves, follow my diet very closely for at least two to eight weeks. If your symptoms improve, your food and beverage toxins are most likely causing your distress.

Examples: My Symptoms

Several symptoms guide me when I search for the foods and beverages causing my symptoms. They include sleep difficulty, paralysis of my intestines, and difficulty remembering names, places, and tasks. I tested many vegetables, including carrots, broccoli, lettuce, and beans; I developed paralysis of my intestines with no bowel sounds or movement with each vegetable trial. The paralysis lasted for three days after I stopped eating the vegetable. A paralyzed intestine feels weird.

After each vegetable trial, my intestine awoke after three days and started working again. Unfortunately, sometimes, only part of the intestine worked; another part didn't. The working part of the intestine kept trying to push material through the sleeping part. The resulting cramping hurt until the entire intestine resumed working and material passed through normally. Instead of intestinal paralysis, a friend suffered painful and noisy intestinal spasms heard across the room that stopped when he changed his diet.

My symptoms also include a sleeping difficulty that troubles me when dementia has a solid hold on me. I sleep for only four hours and wake up feeling tired.

So, paralysis or spasm of the intestine indicates damage to intestinal nerves by dementia. Dementia symptoms could also include poor sleep and the metabolic syndrome I discussed.

Severity of Symptoms

With Mild Dementia Symptoms

I suggest grading your dementia as severe, moderate, or mild. Mild dementia symptoms mean you only need to change your diet slightly to reduce these mild symptoms. First, reduce re-fined sugar in your foods and beverages because these sweet treats are addicting and should go first. Check your food shelves and throw away any foods or beverages labeled with sugar or ingredients that contain sugar.

With Moderate Dementia Symptoms

Moderate symptoms can include:

- Decreased thinking or memory ability.
- A feeling of being unbalanced as you walk.
- Poor sleep.

If you feel these disturbances, reduce your consumption of fructose, MSG, galactose, and citrus acids. Look in my books and search the internet for lists of products containing these chemicals. Dispose of any foods or beverages with added MSG, citrus acids, galactose (dairy), refined sugar. Look especially for anything called flavoring or flavors because this listing most likely means MSG.

With More Severe Dementia Symptoms

With more severe symptoms, you must make a choice. Do you want to continue living with an intact mind and with the freedom and independence that allows you to come and go as you please? To drive north, south, east, or west just because you want to? Or do you want to live in a locked memory unit with somebody to clean your bed when you wake up in the morning? If you vote for clear thinking, freedom, independence, and a clean bed, my diet should help you continue the life you love. We will discuss this diet in the next chapter.

22

My Diet Is the Only Treatment That Reverses Dementia

A Diet to Reverse Disease

Before discussing my diet further, I will explain why my diet is the only treatment that reverses dementia. We have already covered this information, but I wanted to reassemble it into a form that explains why my diet returns you to everyday life with an intact mind. I will start by mentioning treatments that fail to reverse dementia.

Many Treatments Have Failed to Reverse Dementia

There are many treatments for dementia, but they fail to release the sufferer from this brain-stealing disease. One treatment is exercise of the mind and body that keeps your body in tip-top shape. I recommend daily exercise of the mind and body; I walk frequently and exercise my mind daily by studying and writing. However, evidence is scant that exercise of mind or body returns the intelligence stolen by dementia.

Multiple drugs to treat dementia have been studied but all failed to slow or reverse dementia.

Some Modern Diets Slow the Onset Of Dementia

Although drugs and exercise fail to return an alert mind to the afflicted, some diets are partially effective. Many studies show that the Mediterranean, DASH, MIND, and other diets impressively slow the onset of dementia by limiting the consumption of fructose sugar. However, this avoidance does not reverse disease, but they point to a method that does.

Reversing the Dementias by Limiting Food Poisons

As I stated already, reducing the toxins I call the aging chemicals, refined sugar, MSG, citrus, and galactose, is the only treatment that reverses dementia. However, we cannot entirely eliminate these chemicals from our diet nor can we avoid poisons manufactured by food plants because we need these foods to feed us. Fortunately, little proof exists that it is inherently damaging to limit the amount of vegetables and fruits we consume.

What Research Shows

A Contrast With Normally Recommended Food and Beverages

To contrast my diet with the healthy diet advocated by experts, we turn to research published online on March 1, 2021, by the journal *Circulation* that looked at dozens of studies worldwide involving about two million people followed up to thirty years. Doctor Daniel Wang, the lead author, stated that fruits and vegetables are major sources of several nutrients linked to good health, particularly the health of the heart and blood vessels. These nutrients include potassium, magnesium, fiber, and antioxidant plant compounds. The article advocates two servings of fruit and three servings of vegetables per day for a total of five servings daily.

Five Servings a Day

These daily five servings of fruit and vegetables are undoubtedly good advice for people striving for a healthy diet. However, these people do not realize that these diets are not as healthy as they seem; they contain high concentrations of plant toxins and aging chemicals in their fruits and vegetables. Consuming this number of fruits and vegetables significantly impairs mental ability at any age. Adults with dementia who do not limit fructose experience nerve deterioration and suffer increased confusion in stressful situations. Not a good result from a healthy diet.

23

The Heretical Walsh Diet

A Scolding

You already know about dementia and know that no drug treats this disease. The lack of drug treatment suggests that food poisoning causes dementia and not drug-treatable diseases like pneumonia, heart attacks, or depression, although these conditions can accompany dementia.

A Grade School Class Knows the Answer

If grade school children knew that MSG, citrus, and galactose assist the nerve deterioration of fructose and that plant-produced toxins help this deterioration, they would tell you that you can reverse dementia by not eating so much of them. They would be correct. This answer is so apparent that you do not need an advanced education such as an MD or PhD degree to diagnose and treat this simple disease.

Just reduce the toxins consumed daily—a simple, effective, and cheap treatment. I do not know how this simple disease gets by with killing so many people. Even grade school children could learn how to defang this monster snake.

I Don't Know Why

Millions of medical doctors and diet specialists must know this information. However, they seem unaware that home treatment at the dining table can stop it in its tracks. If this is so, why do we still consider dementia such a heartbreaking disease when simple dietary changes prevent dementia's brain deterioration and allow a useful, enjoyable, and long-lived life. These deaths are horrible and a disgrace to the medical profession.

The Chapter on the Diet

Everything I discussed leads inevitably to this chapter on the diet. After all, if I tell you about the dementias but not how to reverse them and recover your mental abilities, I have not helped you. I will show you how I recovered from dementia, and I hope you can do the same. The diet I follow protects me from dementia's destruction, allows me to live many years with the active mind that God (or Nature) gave me.

An Unorthodox Diet

My diet is unorthodox. It is diet heresy. Dictionary.com defines heresy as an opinion or doctrine at variance with the orthodox or accepted doctrine, especially of a church or religious system. Experts praise the Mediterranean, MIND, Mayo Clinic, and other diets, elevating them to sacred status. I do not share this opinion. All "healthy diets" are adequate for people suffering mild dementia, but they do not reverse severe dementia. They short-change these unfortunate people. Although these other diets suggest avoiding fructose and some MSG, MSG in excess is such a poisonous substance that avoiding it should be featured more prominently. Further, these other diets do not avoid galactose, citrus acids, and the food toxins of plants.

How I Discovered These Food Toxins

In this book, I describe a method to discover the toxins that caused dementia. I did not find these toxins by this book's method. I became aware of them because they made so many of my patients sick. So, when I realized that I had dementia, I already had a strong suspicion that these same foods and beverages caused my dementia. I changed my diet to remove the excess aging chemicals and started preparing my food with methods that decreased the toxins of food plants and found that these toxins were indeed at fault.

My Diet Has Similarities to the Carnivore Diet

Both my diet and the carnivore diet rely heavily on meat. A recent article by Miki Ben-Dor and colleagues at Tel Aviv University comments on using a meat-based diet. It concerns research titled "The Evolution of the Human Trophic Level During the Pleistocene" reported in *The American Journal of Physical Anthropology*. The Pleistocene is the Ice Age that lasted from about 2,580,000 to 11,700 years ago. The study presents good evidence that our ancestors ate a meat-based diet with little plant food until they exhausted the supply of large animals. With this supply loss, they turned to our current mixed meat, vegetables, and fruit diet. The study pointed out that we still retain evidence of being well-suited for a meat-based diet.

https://tinyurl.com/yj35hgwg

Describing The Strict Diet

I will now discuss the diet that allowed me to recover from Alzheimer's and Parkinson's dementias. I am not a dietician, so I will describe my diet, not as a dietician but as a doctor specializing in the diseases caused by our diet. That's what I am. You might need a dietician to help you plan your meals.

Vegetables

I already discussed vegetables. Many types of vegetables activate symptoms associated with my dementia, including slowed memory, poor sleep, and paralysis of the intestinal tract. When I search for harmful food chemicals, I must leave my dementia-fighting diet and add vegetables to my meals. To decide whether it worsens my symptoms, I look for my symptoms of poor sleep, paralysis of my intestinal tract, and defects in my memory. If these symptoms appear, I return to my usual diet until the symptoms of deterioration subside and my sleep, intestinal tract, and memory return to functioning normally. Then I retry eating the studied foods— in this example, vegetables—for one to three or more days to determine if my dementia symptoms again deteriorate. Thankfully, after each test, I recovered well.

After following my regular diet for several more days to ensure I was free of dementia, I restarted testing again with another vegetable. It takes a long time to do these diet tests.

Possible Problems With Detection

This complicated and awkward process is the only way that I can identify the foods that worsen my dementia. This process has some defects. During the testing period, I also eat many other foods that may also be causing dementia symptoms, thus making vegetables appear more harmful than they are. I will be returning to re-investigating vegetables to see if the results are still the same and I will report on these trials in the future. In the meantime, I do not include vegetables in my meals. Fortunately, I feel fine without them.

Fruits

I love fruits, so I regret limiting them because of their excess fructose and citrus. I do include wild blueberries in my diet three days a week—Wednesday, Friday, and Sunday—between a half and a full cup of frozen wild blueberries. I call them my sweet treats because the frozen blueberries taste like candy, which I cannot have.

I admit that I miss the delightful taste of excess fructose, MSG, citrus, and galactose-loaded foods and beverages. When I realized that I could include fruits in my diet, I included them in whatever food I prepared. They tasted delightful, like candy. Unfortunately, this excess reactivated my symptoms associated with dementia, including poor sleep, GI paralysis, slipping memory, and rusty thinking skills. I learned that I could only include one pear, peach, or small bowl of wild blueberries per day.

Sometimes I think even this limited amount is too much, and I skip the fruit for a day or more. More about fruits in the future.

Meats

I include varieties of meats in my diet, including chicken, turkey, salmon, trout, beef, and pork, varying them daily to introduce variety into my diet. The meats seem to differ in dementia-causing ability with the least troubling foods eggs and fish, to the most troubling foods chicken and turkey, beef, and pork.

Supplements and Vitamins

Living in the northern United States with little winter sun exposure, I take Vitamin D daily in winter. I suspect it is not necessary during the summer. My use of other vitamins is erratic, and I do not think I can give you a feeling for whether they help or hurt dementia. I know that I must avoid supplements because every supplement I've tried—and I've tried many—causes bleeding from my nose and onto my stools. This bleeding may not be threatening, but I worry that the same bleeding may happen in my brain where it might cause damage, so I do not use any supplements. I have dementia, I do not need further brain damage.

https://tinyurl.com/yjmcathv

Beverages

I drink water and, at times, a small amount of a carefully selected alcoholic drink. I avoid coffee or tea as I suspect that these beverages have the same toxins as other plant-derived foods and beverages. I drink no sweetened beverages, whether artificial or natural sweeteners.

I continue to use the information I obtained from Tom Brady's diet as his Super Bowl wins tell me his diet is super healthy. He drinks many bottles of water daily with potassium and magnesium added for taste. I do the same, suspecting that these taste-lightening chemicals help me. That might be a topic for the next book.

Preparing Meals

The following meals can be prepared in large or small quantities to provide meals for one or more people and for many meals. As our daily meals are similar, all this food is precooked to move as much toxin as possible into the drippings, which I discard.

Being dependent on meat, eggs, and limited fruit for my diet introduces a problem. These foods, especially the meats, have minimal taste unless they are charred or seasoned with one or more of the aging chemicals. As I do not want to feed my dementia, I do not use these taste-increasing chemicals, and charring the meat interferes with poison removal. To introduce a little taste to the food, I mix various cooked meats together.

Preparing Ingredients

The Turkey/Hamburger Ingredient

I use a pressure cooker with a pad of butter and one-half teaspoon of salt dissolved in water with most meat preparations. I place up to six pounds of ground turkey burger and three pounds of ground hamburger in a large bowl with two cups of unsalted water and mix the two types of meat by hand. The water makes the mixing more manageable. You can use all turkey or all hamburger or any combination of these meats in any amount.

I form the meat into small balls to allow heat movement through the meat and place them into the pressure cooker. I use the butter and salt added to the pot to encourage the toxins to dissolve into the water. I add enough water to cover the turkey/ham mixture and pressure cook until it is well cooked—the meat falls off the bone. With a colander, I strain the fluid from the meat and flush the meat with tap water, discarding the fluid and then use or freeze the meat.

Chicken White Meat

The white meat of chicken or turkey (labels clear of toxin) adds flavor to the preparation. Dice (chop the meat into tiny pieces) the white meat and place it in a microwave dish with an enclosed tray that collects the dripping at the bottom. Microwave the meat. I microwave for six minutes, let it cool, and discard the drippings collected in the bottom of the microwave pan, which I suspect contain much of the meat's toxins. I dice the cooked meat further and then use it or freeze it.

Bacon

Select a pound of bacon that has a good meat content. Partially freeze it to make it easier to cut. Dice the bacon and microwave for six minutes and discard the drippings. After it cools, freeze, or use it.

Preparing the Meal

As I mentioned, this meal preparation provides sufficient food for as many meals as you decide. The amount of each ingredient depends on how many people you cook for and the amount of food you want to freeze for later use.

When preparing this meat, I typically place at least six pounds of cooked hamburger/turkey burger into a large bowl.

Add 1 cup of cooked diced white meat.
Add 1 cup of cooked diced bacon.
Crack and add as many eggs as desired.
Mix these ingredients.

Dividing the Meal

Dividing the completed meal preparation into individual portions calls for a judgment on your part. I find that two cups of this mixture satisfy my hunger. You may find this too much or too little, so increase or decrease the amount as you see fit. Divide the servings into individual containers for each future meal and freeze them to thaw and use.

My Usual Meals

The content of my meals is repetitive.

I use a thawed portion of the above mixture for *breakfast*, satisfying my hunger.

My usual *lunch* is canned salmon and some leftover meat from the previous evening.

Evening dinner is fish, fowl, beef, or pork. To prepare the fish, I use a frying pan with the fish lying in a small amount of water, to which I dissolve a small amount of salt and a pad of butter to encourage toxins to migrate into the salt/butter/water. I pressure cook fowl, beef, or pork with water, salt, and butter until the meat separates from the bone.

Taste, Safety, and Cleanliness

You can successfully argue that my diet has little taste. I agree with you. However, I wake up every morning glad I'm alive, thinking clearly, and living independently. I am also delighted that nobody needs to clean the bed after I am out of it. That last thought, the cleaning of the bed, will continue to help me tolerate my diet.

Thank you for reading my book.

There is so much more to tell you, including the possibility that genetic manipulation can restore the protection of the blood–brain barrier, and we can return to eating the poison-filled diet that we call normal. I will discuss that and other issues in the next book, which I will begin soon. Thank you for reading my book, and I hope that everybody suffering from severe dementia sees this book. Let it help them arise in the morning, delighted with the return of their mental ability and meeting the day with a smile.

Addendum

A Presentation

I gave the following presentation that summarizes much of what we discussed in my books. Trying to compress their information into an oral presentation leaves many listeners confused about what I said. With my books, I have more time to present a more complete picture of the cause and treatment of diseases like dementia, and the reader can review my books as necessary to recall individual topics, lessening misunderstanding. Consider these thoughts as you read my presentation and imagine how difficult it must be to understand and treat diseases like dementia after hearing an hour's presentation. Be glad you have the books.

The following is the presentation:

The dementias, including Alzheimer's, Parkinson's, and Lewy body, are simple to explain and understand. Poisons, also called toxins, are in all of our foods. The body protects our brains from these toxins, but aging degrades this shield, and we suffer from dementia. Diet change can lead to recovery. Now, that is a simple explanation, easy to understand.

Or perhaps it isn't. Too many questions remain unanswered. For instance, what makes diets unhealthy? What are toxins, and how do they contaminate foods? What foods do they contaminate? What protects the brain from these poisons, and what degrades this protection? To reverse dementia, what foods and beverages should be limited or avoided?

Seemingly healthy diets promote foods that are considered healthy, such as leafy greens and fresh fruit. However, these foods do not make a diet healthy; reducing the toxins in the foods and beverages make a diet healthy. To consume a healthy diet, dieters must reduce disease-promoting toxins to a level that does not destroy brains.

What foods contain these toxins? All foods contain them. To survive, all plants produce toxins to defend themselves from the mold, insects, and animals that want to eat them. You see the effects of this poison in trees; when the poisons are ineffective, tragedies like Dutch elm disease and chestnut blight strike, and trees die. Similarly, food plants also produce defensive toxins, and the plants die when the toxins fail to protect, as seen in the Irish potato famine. We eat these poisons when we eat the plants. The meat of plant predators like cattle and pigs contain these plant poisons from their food, and we consume the toxins when we eat meat.

A barrier called the blood–brain barrier protects the brain of all creatures with nervous systems from these toxins, beginning with jellyfish and ending with humans. However, for various reasons, the barrier deteriorates, allowing toxins to enter the brain, destroy its nerves, and bring on dementia. We can reverse dementia by preparing the diet so that less poison flows to the brain.

My books tell my story of how I recovered from dementia. I did not develop this approach by myself. The people suffering from the diseases caused by our foods and beverages are the foremost authority on their conditions, and they helped me. Being affected by these poisons, they understand them. I often considered their thoughts mistaken until I discovered that they were not mistaken. They were right!

For instance, children suffering red, itchy rashes taught me that a citrus burn of the skin causes a common skin rash called eczema or atopic dermatitis. I could not believe that until I saw that reducing or removing acids from the diet of eczema sufferers often relieves these uncomfortable rashes. Another example: A dear friend taught me that exaggerated reactions to MSG frequently cause painful migraine and cluster headaches, a cause still little appreciated.

You do not need an advanced academic degree to understand the dementias. The concepts are simple, as are the various factors that cause this disease.

If you do not have dementia, you do not need to follow my path to health. However, when you face a stressful experience that demands that your thinking be razor-sharp, going on a toxin-reduced diet for several weeks should help you. You may be eating foods and drinking beverages with significant amounts of toxins that you can eliminate without undue distress. Avoiding these toxins helps thinking, self-confidence and IQ, even in people free of dementia.

If your dementia is mild, you may need to change my diet only minimally. With more advanced dementia, you need to follow my diet more closely to see if it helps you and continue to follow it if it does. Perhaps your thinking and planning have deteriorated so much that your family is threatening to take your keys away, or they are checking out possible openings in a memory unit. These actions may stimulate you to follow the diet closely. Allowing dementia to progress can only end your liberty. If my diet helps you, it might be able to preserve your freedom.

I hope I have opened your eyes to the threats to your health posed by our poisonous diet. Please tell me your thoughts after you read my book. To do this, leave me a comment on my website, drwewalsh.com, or on my book's page on Amazon; look for the book's name, *Escape from Dementia*, and my name, William Emmett Walsh, MD. Click on "Write a customer review" and leave your note or your review. I will learn from you as I learned from my patients, and I will be grateful that you shared your insights.